POWER POSITIONS

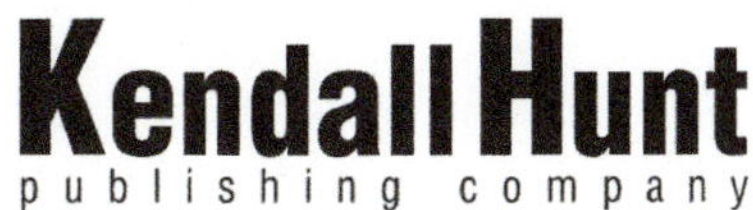

POWER POSITIONS

Championship Prescriptions for Ultimate Sports Performance

by Andrea Hudy

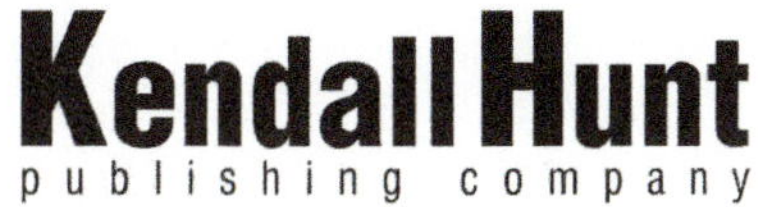

Cover image courtesy of Kansas Athletics, Inc.

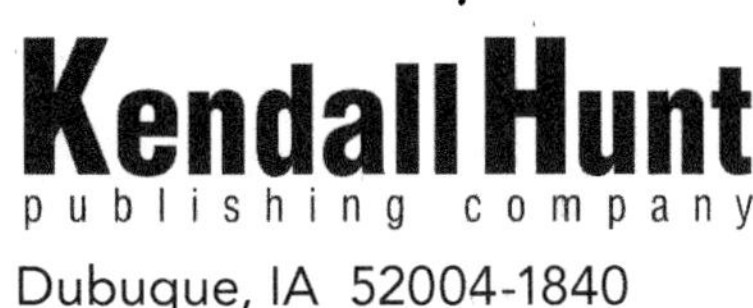

Dubuque, IA 52004-1840

ISBN 978-1-4652-6068-0

Printed in the United States of America

CONTENTS

Strength:

1. the quality or state of beingstrong; bodily or muscular power; vigor.
2. mental power, force, or vigor.
3. moral power, firmness, or courage.
4. power by reason of influence, authority, resources, numbers, etc.

-Websters

ACKNOWLEDGEMENTS

Power Positions has been a work in progress not only since my career as a sports performance coach began, but from the start of my active lifestyle. This book has been made possible through the unwavering love and support from my family and friends. Having come from a background of teachers and competitive athletes, the only thing I have known is to give my best effort. My parents and older siblings coached me through the first phase of my life—"Growing up." They provided a foundation of dedication, commitment, hard work, competition, persistence, and strength. My parents showed me the true value of an ability to make a connection and teach someone, while my siblings forced me to find the competitive drive that is so prevalent throughout my life.

As an athlete, my greatest influences were Betsy Mason, my high school volleyball coach; Janice Kruger, who provided me with the opportunity to compete as a volleyball player at the University of Maryland; and Susie Homan, who helped me thrive as a collegiate student-athlete and adult. These mentors have taught me the value of relationships and coaching. Coach Russ Rose at Penn State University and Laurie Lokash at Slippery Rock University were also vital members of developing my sports career. Even though I did not have the opportunity to play for them in college, their coaching standards influence me to this day.

The progress I have made in my career has not come without help. None of my accomplishments would have been possible without the coaches who have so graciously embraced me. Among these amazing coaches are Bill Self, Jim Calhoun, Geno Auriemma, Bonnie Henrickson, Katie O'Connor, Chris Dailey, Joe Dooley, and the many great coaches at the University of Kansas. Equally important are the administrators who have provided the opportunities to help us succeed along the way: Sheahon Zenger, Lew Perkins, Jeff Hathaway, and Sean Lester.

Dr. William Kraemer, Dr. Andrew Fry, Dr. Phil Wagner, and the National Strength and Conditioning Association (NSCA) continuously provide opportunity to learn new things and inspire me to never waver from the developmental process. As humans, we strive to know the truth about the world we live in; these people have dedicated their lives to searching for the quantification and validation behind what is taught on a daily basis.

I would be lost without the assistance and support of our staff at the University of Kansas: Glenn Cain, Luke Bradford and Patricia Dietz. They have helped facilitate and organize the daily goals that make everything possible. I will always pull for our staff because I know how much they persist to make things happen for the great athletes and coaches in our athletic department. Many of my assistants have moved up to become a head coach at another organization. Though we no longer work together on a daily basis, we are still colleagues and friends.

Jerry Martin, my mentor from the University of Connecticut, has had the greatest influence on my development as a sports performance coach. My philosophy embodies many of his ideals and I will forever have respect for him.

Ann and Steve Hertzog, who have helped make this book what it is visually, deserve an enormous amount of credit. They are more than just amazing professionals, they are amazing people. I can't express the amount of support they have given me in the production of *Power Positions*.

The athletes are the reason I wake up in the morning. I entered this profession to influence young athletes and help them become stellar people. These athletes have gone on to not only be winners in sport, but winners in life.

Obviously, I cannot specifically acknowledge each individual who has influenced me as there have been a countless number of people who have supported me. Without the help of each and every one of them, things would either have not gotten done, or would have been very difficult to accomplish alone. I am extremely grateful for all who have helped me along this journey.

I am excited for the future as I look forward to continued growth and development. With the amount of support I have in my corner, it is impossible to truly fail. A wise friend once said, "Success is making the most of every opportunity that is presented."

www.AndreaHudy.com

PHOTO CREDITS

Cover: Ben McLemore, 7th overall pic in 2013 NBA draft
by Jeff Jacobsen, Kansas Athletics Inc.

Action shots by Jeff Jacobsen, Kansas Athletics Inc.
and Steven Hertzog

xii Courtesy of Tami Hoffman.

1, 9, 13, 14, 16-17 (bottom row), 19, 23, 27, 29, 37, 39, 45, 47, 49, 51, 69, 75, 81, 89 © Kansas Athletics, Inc. Reprinted by permission.

5, 7, 11, 15, 16-17 (top row), 18, 21, 54, 61, 62, 71, 73, 87, back cover: Steven Hertzog

12, 53, 64, 65, 67, 76, 90 Courtesy of the author.

70 Courtesy of Danielle Meyer, Canadian Sport for Life.

EDITORS: Ann Frame Hertzog & Steven Hertzog

CREATIVE DIRECTOR: Ann Frame Hertzog

In loving memory of Mary Hudy,
my strength.

To: Dad, Mike, Beth, Susan, Tom and Friends
Appreciate Everything!

INTRODUCTION

Experience is the best teacher.

Throughout my career I have been fortunate to work with and gain knowledge from many coaches and athletes who are at the top of their respective sports. I have worked with award winning strength and conditioning coaches, Hall of Fame basketball coaches, and future Hall of Fame coaches and athletes. The number and type of athletes that I have coached also continues to grow: Cross-country runners, football players, Olympic athletes, and professional athletes (37 NBA players and 21 WNBA players, and a few NFL athletes). I have garnered nine NCAA Division I National Championships (three men's basketball, five women's basketball, and one men's soccer) and many more Big 12, Big East, and Atlantic Coast Conference Championships in all sports.

I was humbled to be the recipient of the 2012 National Strength & Conditioning Coach of the Year Award from the National Strength and Conditioning Association. I am cognizant of the fact that the experiences I have had, the great coaches that have been my mentors, and the staff I have worked with have all helped mold my philosophies and insights as a leader and a coach. I have partnered with Dr. Phil Wagner with Sparta Science and it has opened my eyes to defining and assessing movement in a more focused way. I hope to share these methods with you in the following chapters as you read *Power Positions: Championship Prescriptions for Ultimate Sports Performance.*

Power Positions: Championship Prescriptions for Ultimate Sports Performance is a practical science-based training guide to increase athletic performance. There are millions of people who participate in sports:

1. Young athletes competing for a spot on a competitive team
2. High school athletes competing for college scholarships
3. College athletes who have limited access to a performance coach
4. Adults who play recreational sports who want to stay healthy

All of these athletes, no matter the level, want to increase performance and be the most competitive they can be, while others want to simply stay healthy and away from injury. The training programs that are discussed in this book are neither age or gender specific; they are for EVERYONE.

An athlete is an athlete, but the position in the sport you play is where the difference lies in terms of specific strength development, sequencing of force production, and training. These differences are especially important if the athlete plays more than one sport. The multi-sport athlete should understand the qualities that are required for various sport positions. Knowing what specific movement skills are required for similar positions in other sports can facilitate an athlete's decision in what positions to play.

There are three types of positions that emphasize three different types of training:

1. **Lateral moving or reactive athlete**
2. **Rotational athlete**
3. **Linear moving, speed athlete, or timing athlete**

Each position has a specific training program that emphasizes specific movement patterns because different sport positions require a different order or sequence of force production. Force production is the ability to apply force into the ground through your body to create movement. The series of muscle contractions from the ground is called sequencing and it is an important concept for everyone to understand.

For example, a defensive back in football would be suited for basketball or jumping events in track because the athlete uses similar force production when reacting to the ground for lateral and/or vertical movement. On the other hand, an outside receiver in football may be better suited to sprint for track because their force production is similar because they are sprinting to reach top speed in a predetermined path. A tennis player would be a good golfer because of the similar ability to create rotational power through mobility in the torso.

I consider the training programs that are specific to an athlete's movement sequence as exercise prescriptions. I call them exercise prescriptions - just like a doctor's medical prescription for a patient is specific to keep them healthy, a performance coach's exercise prescription is specific to the athlete's movement patterns. If an athlete plays a position that they are not trained to play, then performance will not be optimal and the opportunity for injury will increase.

Exercise prescription by position is a concept that I have learned by working with Dr. Wagner of Sparta Science. Dr. Wagner studies the ground reaction forces of elite athletes and statistically proves an athlete's force production sequence as it relates to high performance and injury prevention. This book will guide you through important concepts regarding force production, movement, and efficiency. Another important concept that is discussed is that more muscle is not always better, in fact, too much muscle mass, can hinder movement and decrease efficiency. Power Positions explains this very important concept.

Power Positions also presents athletes with a necessary understanding of movement principles and the awareness of developmental ages of trainability. Knowledge of these factors, along with the understanding of how to start training and what exercises to utilize, will help to maximize the athlete's potential, develop confidence, and decrease the odds of injury. The workouts provided are easy to read and implement and are differentiated for varying ability levels. Readers will learn about goal setting, programming, and the use of non-linear periodization as a framework for individual or team workouts. Non-linear programming uses the time of year (in season, off season, etc.) or simply how the athlete feels on a given day as a guide for differentiating programming.

Even the most elite athlete, EVERY great athlete, was once a beginner. Starting as a blank slate, athletes are slowly molded by the experiences they are provided. Today's athletes no longer need to be the product of a trial and error mentality of training. The workouts provided are position specific and can be utilized by young athletes, high school athletes, college athletes, adults who play recreational sports, the coach looking for direction with a team, and the more experienced athlete wanting a more advanced prescription.

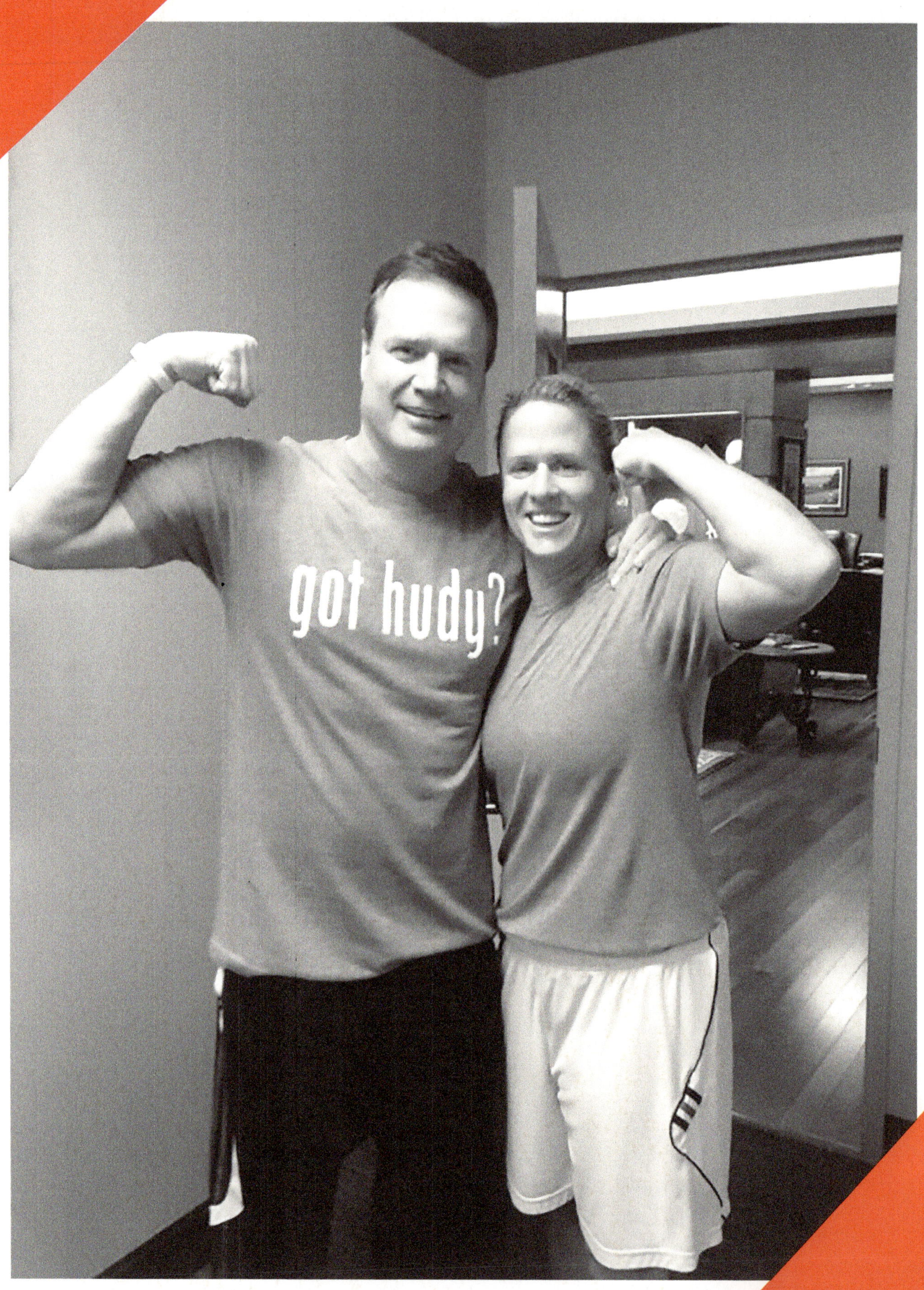

Bill Self and me

FOREWORD

In 2004, I began the search for a new performance coach for our men's basketball program. I lined up several qualified candidates to interview for the position; all of which were men. Our then Athletic Director, Lew Perkins, insisted that I add one more candidate to the list.

"A woman? A woman... to be a men's basketball strength coach? Who does that?!"

Lew didn't budge, and again insisted that I just listen to what she had to say.

I granted Lew the request and sat down with Andrea. She had worked with the tenacious coaching greats, Auriemma and Calhoun, at UConn. They had just won the NCAA Championship...both men's and women's programs...so I knew that they were doing something right.

However, I still wasn't convinced. Hiring a woman, even from a recruiting standpoint, could be a huge risk. I offered the position to another candidate.

He decided he didn't want to move to Kansas. Back to square one. I was running out of time.

Andrea's experience and her obvious passion for teaching athletes was something I couldn't deny and that stuck with me. Despite my hesitation, I decided to go ahead and offer her the position on a probationary status...one year and then we'd reassess and see how things were going.

.....Ten years later, I can still say that it was one of the best hiring decisions I've made.

Andrea has a gift in the ability to maximize a guy's athletic potential. While many performance coaches are the stereotypical, rough, demanding, and gruff kind of coach; Andrea is more of a two-dimensional coach. Don't get me wrong, she'll demand more out of our guys than they know they're capable of... but Andrea has the other side, the ability to establish genuine relationships with our guys. In some, she fills a sort of mother figure role. She cares enough about them as individuals to do whatever it takes to help them become the best athlete and person they can be.

Andrea not only demands the best of our athletes, but also of herself and the program. She is hungry for perfection. As a result, Andrea is always refining herself as a coach. She seeks to balance proven best practices with the latest in cutting edge technology. Her passion is why our strength program is arguably the best in the country. Her science based approach combined with the latest technology and software puts our athletes at the forefront of performance training.

I once worried that having a female strength coach would be a detriment to recruiting. As it turns out, Andrea is one of the reasons WHY athletes decide to come to Kansas. Her results based programming gets our guys ready for the next level.

-Bill Self, NCAA Championship Coach, 10 Straight Big 12 Titles

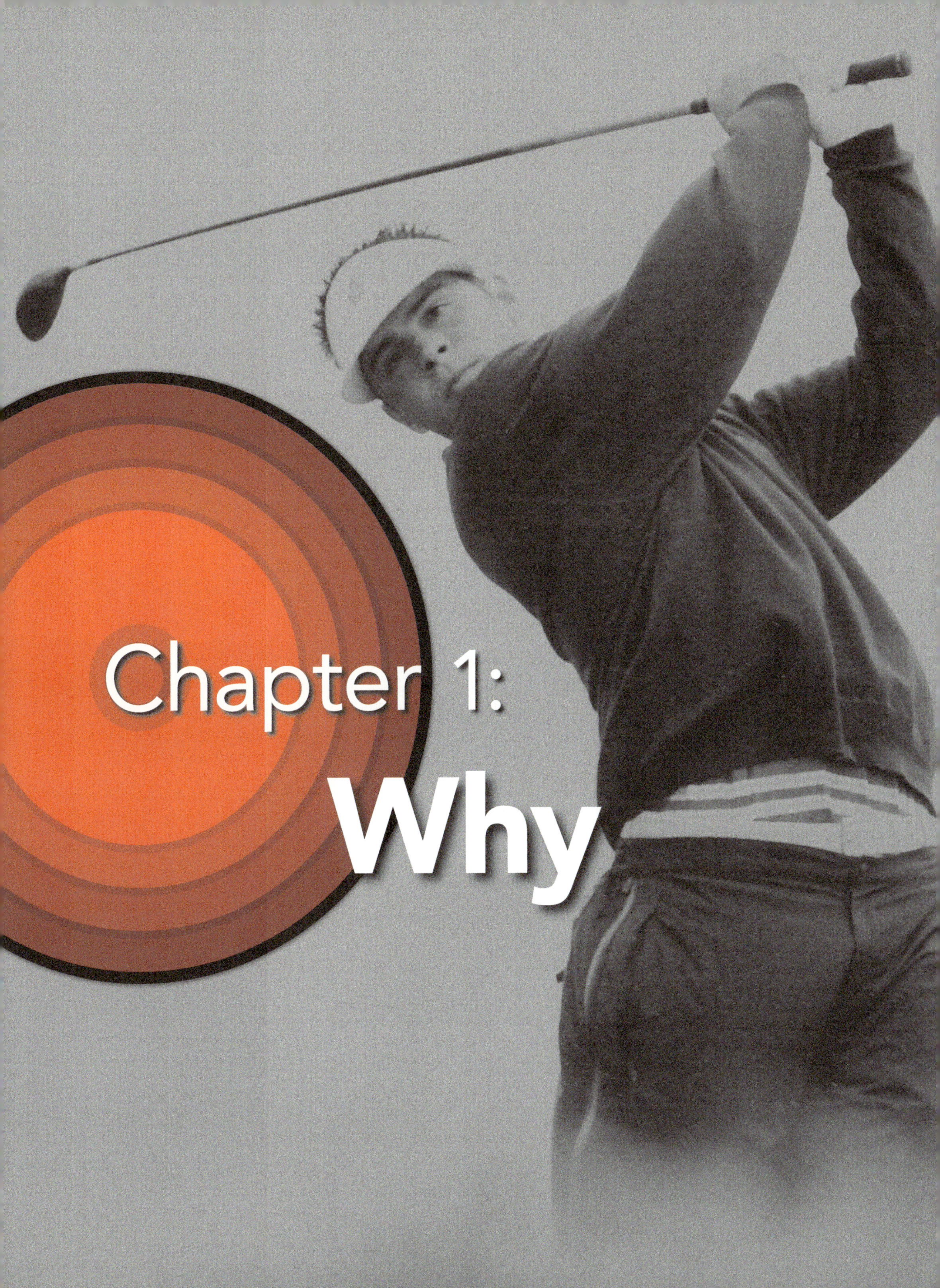

Chapter 1: Why

SECTION 1: Movement Qualities

Human movement is about function

Athletes who participate in different sports may have different backgrounds; so, as a performance coach, it is important to develop a solid foundation of basic performance skills: running, skipping, hopping, jumping, squatting, lunging, twisting, etc. Most athletes who I have come across have little experience with a comprehensive training program before they arrive at college, so it is important for me to share some basic principles and programs for those who want to train.

The first day I meet an athlete, they are treated as though they have never had any type of training. This happens for many reasons, some of which are worth mentioning:

- I don't know their true training background.
- The athletes don't speak the performance language that we do, so we must teach them our language.
- Although there is a full physical completed before they start to train, I don't have a great concept of their mobility and/or limitations due to past experiences and old/new injuries.

I look at different abilities that our athletes have when it comes to movement. Human movement is about function: Functions such as walking, running, jumping, squatting, lunging, shuffling, twisting, turning, or any combination thereof. Most functions can be generalized into the following three movement categories:

1. LOAD

The **ability to decelerate or control the body against gravity through anterior chain strength** is the ability to LOAD. As athletes brake into the ground, they are using the muscular system's ability to stretch then potentially snap back (EXPLODE) with strength like a tight elastic rubber band. When we walk, it is low intensity cyclic deceleration (load) and acceleration (explode) of the body against gravity. When we run and jump, the intensity is simply greater. Reactive athletes, such as basketball players, defensive backs, long jumpers, and high jumpers who change direction quickly (vertical, lateral), have to have an ability to load. Also, someone like an offensive lineman who has to slow something down should have great deceleration qualities.

2. EXPLODE

The **ability to create strength through muscle stiffness and brace against forces** is an ability to EXPLODE. Explode comes after load. The more efficient the athlete, the easier it becomes to load into the ground with greater explosion or strength off of the ground. Muscle stiffness can be trained with short ballistic, fast contractions that do not require full ranges of motion; but the athlete should be able to maintain strength or stiffness in a full range of motion. When we jump, change direction, or brace against contact of an object or person, we create stiffness. Reactive athletes and athletes who can accelerate aggressively have the ability to create high EXPLODE which creates greater movement efficiency (jump higher and run faster). Athletes who have a low EXPLODE have mobility in the torso (lack of stiffness or compliance). This allows them the ability to produce great ranges of motion in order to create rotatory power.

3. DRIVE

The **ability to overcome gravity to reach and maintain maximum speed through compliant muscular contractions in the posterior chain** is referred to as DRIVE. Compliant muscular contractions can be trained with long healthy contractions through a complete range of motion. Athletes who reach top speed and use momentum (sprinters, receivers, outside hitters) to their advantage, or athletes who have to push an object (defensive lineman) all have to have great abilities to DRIVE. These athletes may appear smooth or fluid and may use a timing ability while performing a skill.

These abilities are important to me because not only do they make sense, they are abilities that Dr. Wagner at Sparta Science has proven to be the main characteristics of proper sequencing in different sport positions: Load, explode, drive.

Ground reaction forces are the foundation for movement. These are the forces generated by the athlete as a consequence of contact with the ground.

Imagine trying to play your position on ice? There is no way you could maximally brake, sprint, or throw without a pair of ice skates to provide better ground reaction forces. The only way that an athlete could perform a basic movement skill is if you gain better contact with the surface with a pair of ice skates.

When you began playing positions in soccer, softball, or basketball, what was the first purchase you or your parents made? Most of the time, the first purchase was a pair of sport-specific shoes. This is done so that the athlete can create better ground reaction forces to move more effectively.

Some athletic shoes have cleats for better acceleration/ deceleration on grass or dirt, some shoes have more lateral support to assist in lateral reactivity, and some have rubber soles to grip the court. Having the proper footwear allows us to have better contact with the ground. That is why we assess and train movement from the ground up, starting with the feet through the body. Picture a volleyball or basketball player wiping the dirt off of the bottom of their shoes with their hands or with a sticky slipknot pad? It is the same reason why football players change their cleats and baseball players knock the dirt off of the bottom of their shoes. Track athletes also change the size of their cleats depending on the surface that they are competing on. Soccer players have indoor and outdoor shoes because the surfaces are different. This is done to increase the quality and/or reactability of movement with the ground or increase ground reaction forces. Even the surface of a diving board is rough. It just makes sense that our athlete's movement is assessed and trained from the ground up by utilizing ground-based training principles.

LOAD
or The Ability to Decelerate

Deceleration occurs when force is absorbed, controlled, or something is slowed down or stopped in the direction of movement. This happens when we control flexion of ankle, knee, and hip (triple flexion) and create some level of trunk/torso stiffness to absorb momentum. We train deceleration when we protect and control our bodies against gravity. Activities like controlling running down a hill, jumping off a box, or jumping down steps train anterior chain movements.

Cars are great decelerators because of the great braking systems, but they are not great accelerators when compared to jet planes or boats. Cars make quick turns after braking which make them reactive. Defense-minded athletes, like basketball players, tend to be great reactive decelerators because they are braking all the time in order to change direction whether it's laterally or vertically. Defensive backs are great decelerators because they have to react to the receiver's running pattern. When we compare lateral or reactive athletes to linear athletes, lateral or reactive athletes should have greater anterior chain strength and reactive stiffness (strength).

Everyone can relate to driving down the road and a squirrel runs in the way. The squirrel gets startled by the oncoming car and reactively dodges left, right, left, and right again before it figures out which direction to accelerate. A predatory cheetah is more reactive than a kangaroo because it has front legs to use in deceleration and locomotion. These front legs can act as brakes to help change direction or decelerate. If one compares a two-legged animal like a human to a four-legged animal like a dog, the human rarely ever catches the dog because the dog has much better reactive skills than the human. The dog has back legs for acceleration, but more importantly, front legs to facilitate with deceleration.

In the following picture, the athletes are showing that jumping downstairs is a good way to train anterior chain strength and deceleration capabilities. Controlling the landing from a jump is a great way for basketball athletes and lateral or reactive athletes to train proper sequencing when landing or stopping before acceleration.

Anterior Chain — Generally involved in controlling deceleration of the body against gravity. The link from the ground up from the foot through the mobile ankle (eccentric calf contraction), stable knee (eccentric quadriceps contraction), mobile hip (eccentric gluteus group contraction), and stable lumbar.

Eccentric Muscle Contraction — Force or tension developed in the muscle as it lengthens.

Muscle Stiffness — when a muscle is tight and rigid. Stiff muscles resist deformation in response to an applied force.

Reactive — highly responsive to a stimulus.

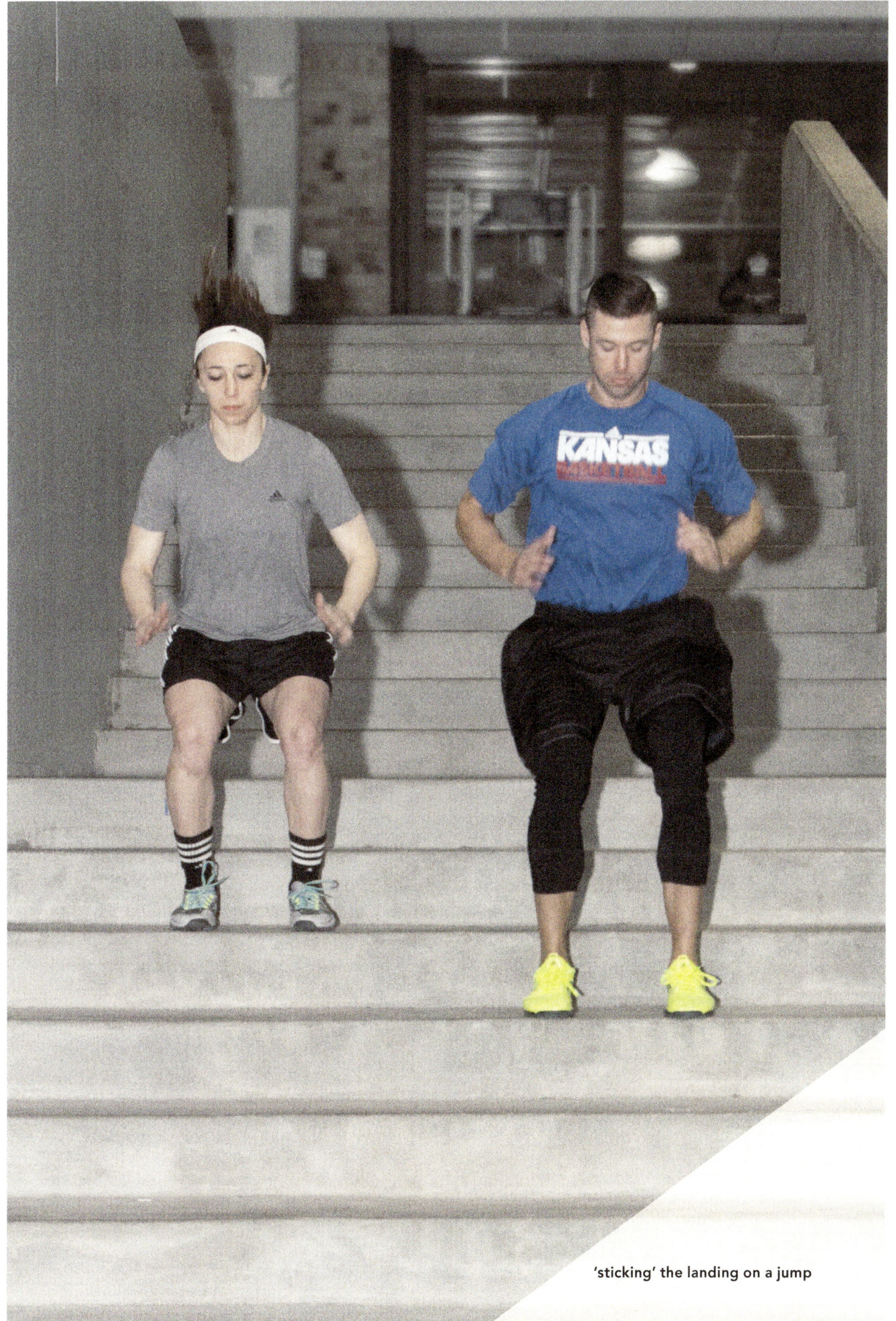

'sticking' the landing on a jump

EXPLODE
or The Ability to Brace or Create Stiffness or Strength

Stiffness provides strength and support, like the Golden Gate Bridge. It is a strong bridge that holds two points of land together. It effectively carries enormous amounts of force that cars and trucks produce in order to get across the water. Can you think of the stiff and erect posture that your coaches/ teachers/trainers always reminded you to correct? When I think of stiffness, I think of the amount of strength to brace in an individual's trunk. Like a bridge, it supports and holds the upper body and the lower body together. Linebackers, defensive backs, rugby players, jumpers, and basketball players have to have a great ability to brace against contact and/or react to move vertically or laterally. These athletes have the ability to create enormous amounts of force in order to move a rigid object (the body or trunk) quickly, without losing stiffness to increase movement efficiency. Exercises such as depth jumps (shock method), plyometrics, squats, dead lifts, lateral agility drills, one sided farmer's walks, wide-grip pull-ups and all posturing movements increase muscular stiffness in the torso. These exercises are intense and ultimately train protective skills from contact or falling.

For a rotatory athlete (golfer, pitcher), this quality of movement is relatively low, but for good reason. The torso should be compliant so when creating rotatory power, it can create a large range of motion in order to 'whip' the object the athlete is hitting or throwing.

When you were younger, do you remember jumping off high ledges? There was probably a point where you stopped because you knew if you went any higher you were going to get hurt. These types of exercises increase muscle stiffness.

Think of car suspension springs; they are tight, stiff and handle a lot forces. When threatened, a snake coils and becomes stiff for an attack in order to become quick and reactive; otherwise it is very compliant in its movement.

Triple Flexion – The coordinated flexion of the ankle, knee, and hip that occurs during deceleration in movements like the stance phase in running and landing from a jump.

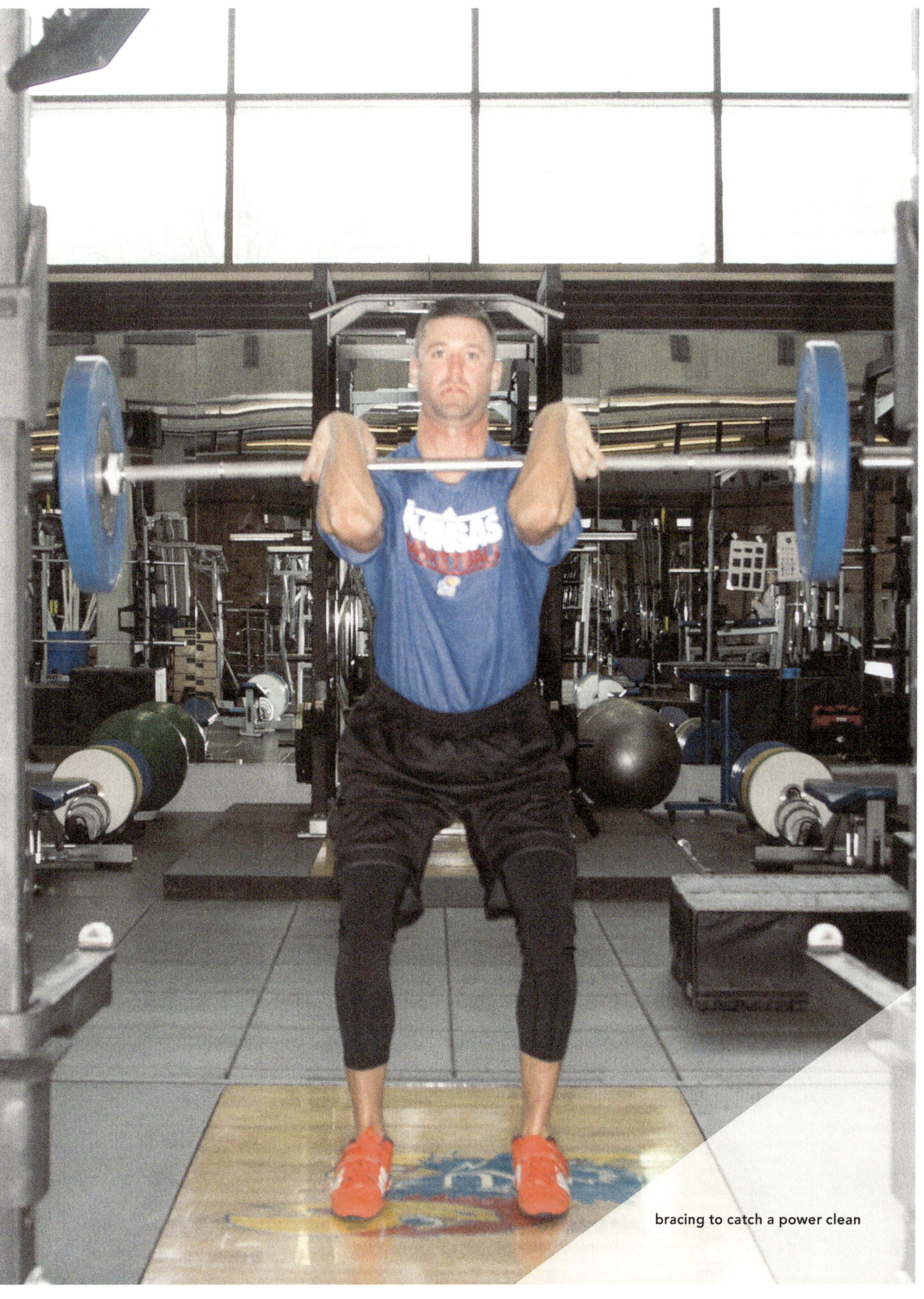

bracing to catch a power clean

DRIVE
or The Ability to Maintain Speed with Compliant Muscular Contractions

Drive is the ability to maintain speed through compliant contractions in the posterior chain. Compliant muscular contractions can be trained with contractions through a full range of motion. Athletes who reach top speed and use momentum (sprinters, outside receivers, safeties, outside hitters) to their advantage, or athletes who have to push an object (defensive linemen) all have to have great abilities to push through or use momentum to their advantage.

In the example of locomotion, extension of ankle, knee, and hip (triple extension) against the ground will cause movement. Generally speaking, any time we overcome gravity, we are primarily utilizing the gluteus maximus, hamstring group, and calves or the posterior chain. We can train the posterior chain with squatting, lunging, weightlifting, sprints, plyometrics or anything that can assist in training triple extension.

Jet planes and boats are great examples of objects that reach top speed and keep momentum; but these objects lack decelerating abilities. They do not have strong enough braking mechanisms to stop their own mass quickly. Athletes who have great drive know the target they are aiming for so they know where they are running. There is no reactive deceleration in running a straight line at top speed. Sprinters and offensive minded athletes such as outside receivers are great accelerators who tend to have lower reactive capabilities. Think of a track sprinter. Sometimes at the end of a race, there is a mat for the athletes to run into to help them stop.

A Kangaroo has a great ability for speed. Kangaroos have hugely developed hind legs (posterior chain) and small 'arms' that are not used for braking or changing direction.

Compliance facilitates movement, like a rope bridge between two mountains. The bridge holds two points of land together. As compared to the stiff Golden Gate Bridge, this bridge requires movement. It's not as strong as the Golden Gate, yet withstands wind and other environmental forces, so it needs to have movement to keep its integrity. It also efficiently holds the force of the people walking across it. Increased compliance provides greater functional range of motion with less stiffness. I often think of an ice skater that uses long lateral strides while speeding around a track or athletes on the kickoff team in American football (usually when the football is kicked into the end zone for a touchback these athletes continue to run to the back of the end zone).

People who perform yoga regularly do not hurry through the movements; that would go against the purpose of the exercise. The focus is on long, healthy muscular contractions from complete flexion to complete extension or vice versa. These types of exercises decrease stiffness. Compliance and mobility are what make baseball pitchers, tennis players, and golfers great at their sports. Fluid and long (not stiff) throws/swings specifically through the torso make them different from other athletes who require stiffness for intense reacting or running.

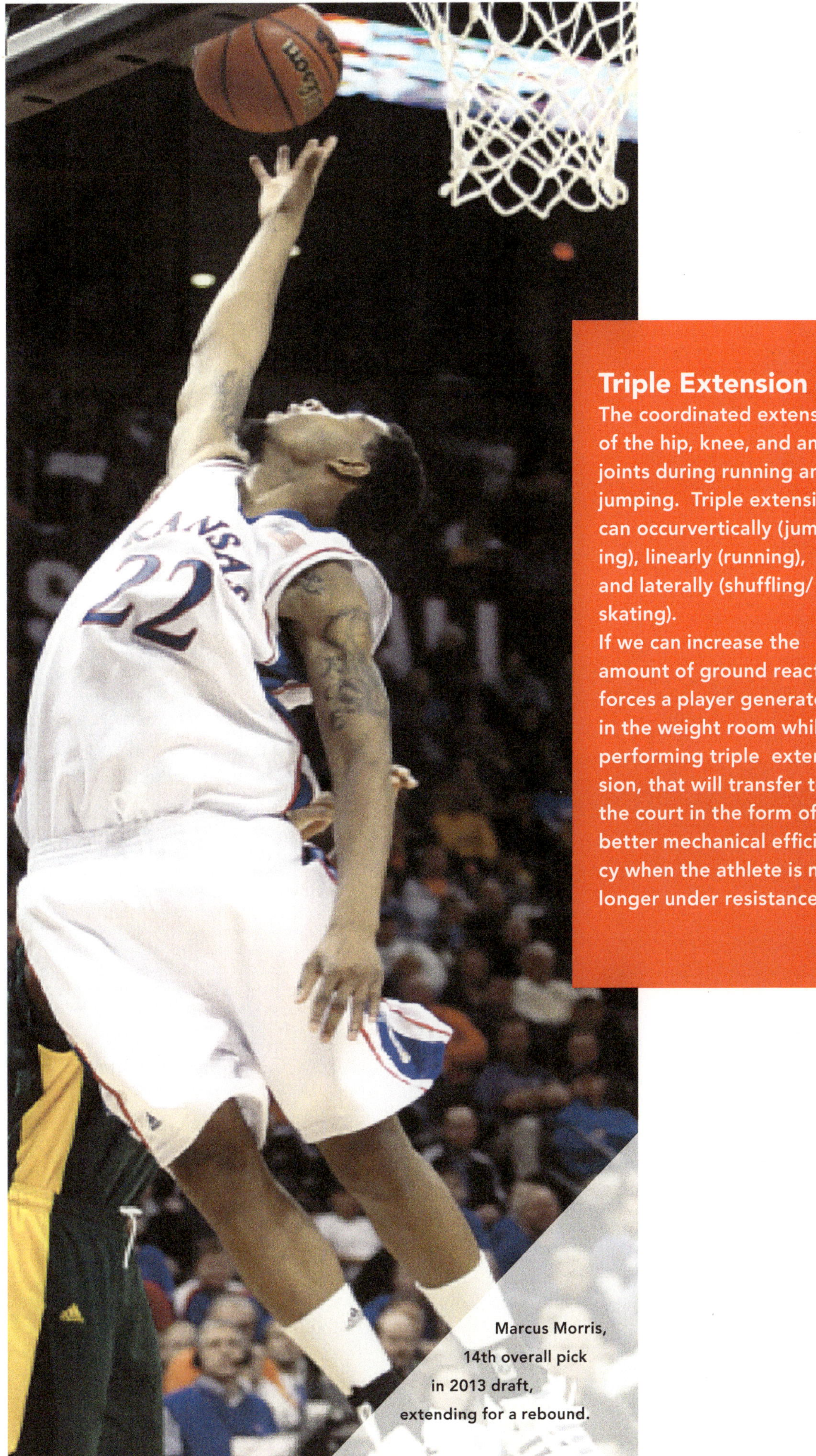

Marcus Morris, 14th overall pick in 2013 draft, extending for a rebound.

Triple Extension –

The coordinated extension of the hip, knee, and ankle joints during running and jumping. Triple extension can occurvertically (jumping), linearly (running), and laterally (shuffling/skating).

If we can increase the amount of ground reaction forces a player generates in the weight room while performing triple extension, that will transfer to the court in the form of better mechanical efficiency when the athlete is no longer under resistance.

When I think of mobility, I think of a motor cross motorcycle. Something that accelerates up a hill to overcome gravity then twists and turns in the air and decelerates when it hits the ground to finish the trick. I also think of street motocycle that twists and turns in the street or highway to get in and out of traffic. When I think of compliance, I think of a slinky, it is mobile and you can move it easily like a snake slithering through the grass or one that is resting on a rock. It's not stiff and coiled for attack, but it is bent and relaxed.

Posterior Chain — Generally involved in acceleration of the body to overcome gravity. The link from the ground up from the foot through the mobile ankle (concentric calf contraction), stable knee (concentric quadriceps contraction), mobile hip (concentric gluteus group contraction), and stable lumbar.

Concentric Muscle Contraction — Force or tension developed in the muscle as it shortens.

Muscle Compliance — When a muscle is flexible and cooperative. Compliant muscles submit and mold to an applied force.

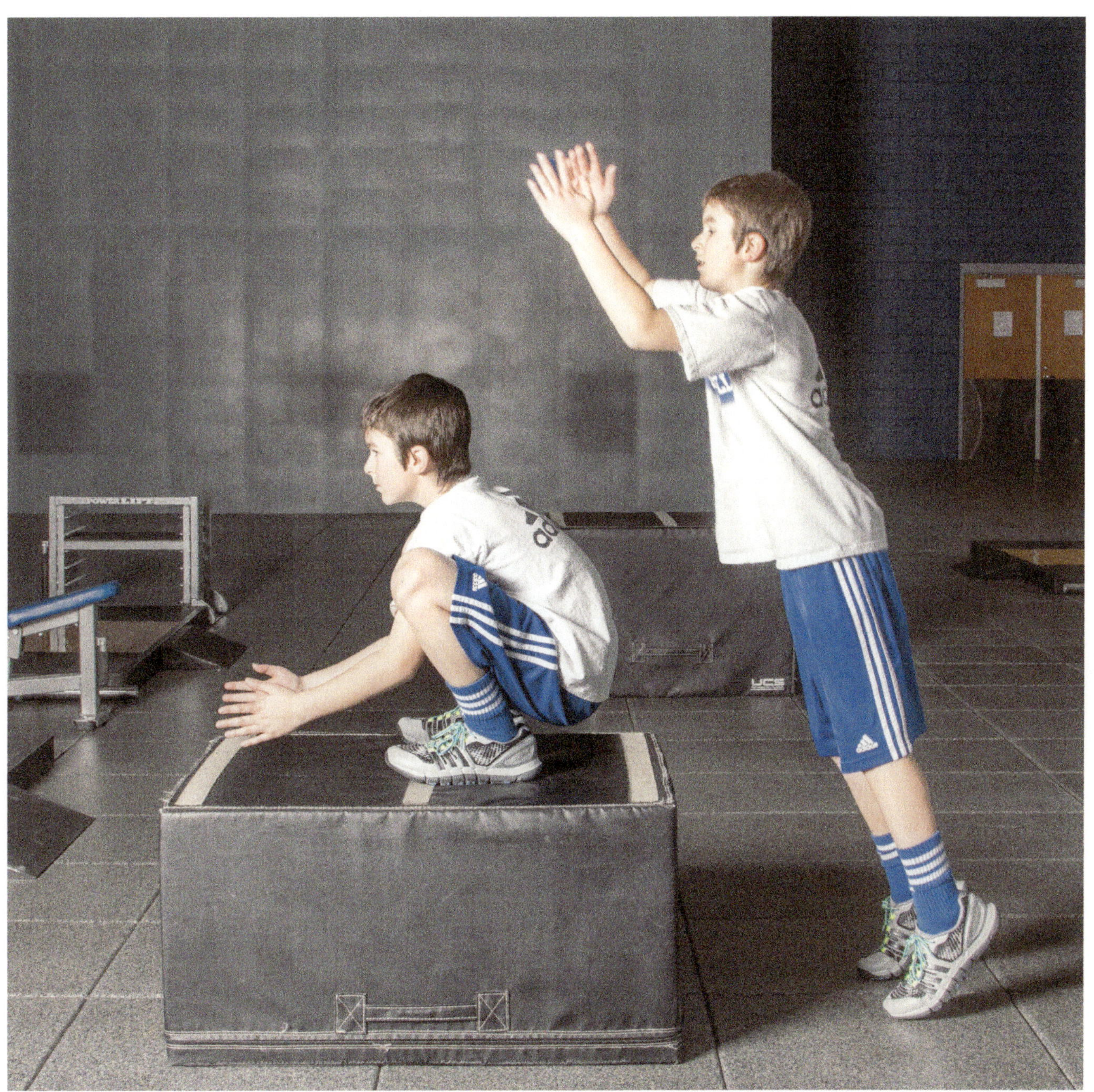

Triple extension in a jump and mobility in a full squat landing.

Conclusion

These three abilities generalize movement patterns that occur in athletics. These abilities interplay with each other as force production becomes specific to a certain skill. Every athlete should train the gamut of these abilities, but certain patterns that are specific to the position played should be trained in order to excel. A performance coach can enhance or actually diminish these abilities through the exercise prescriptions. Each one of these movement patterns requires specific sequencing of muscle recruitment for force production and injury prevention. If an athlete requires a skill that they are not prepared to perform, this puts them at a greater risk of injury.

Andrew Wiggins was a special athlete at Kansas because he not only had a great ability to brace and react quickly, but also an ability to be mobile through full ranges of motion with long healthy compliant muscular contractions. He has the complete range of movement abilities and could utilize a specific ability at the right moment for what needed to be performed on the court at a specific time. Many of our top athletes have these abilities. They are high performers; but, most importantly, they stay healthy.

A coach or athlete should examine what is primarily required for the sport, position, or event:

1. LOAD: Is deceleration required for the skill?
2. EXPLODE: Does the position require reactive change of direction for defense, great posture to be an efficient runner on offense, or fluid movements for rotational power?
3. DRIVE: Is top speed, momentum, or timing required for the skill?

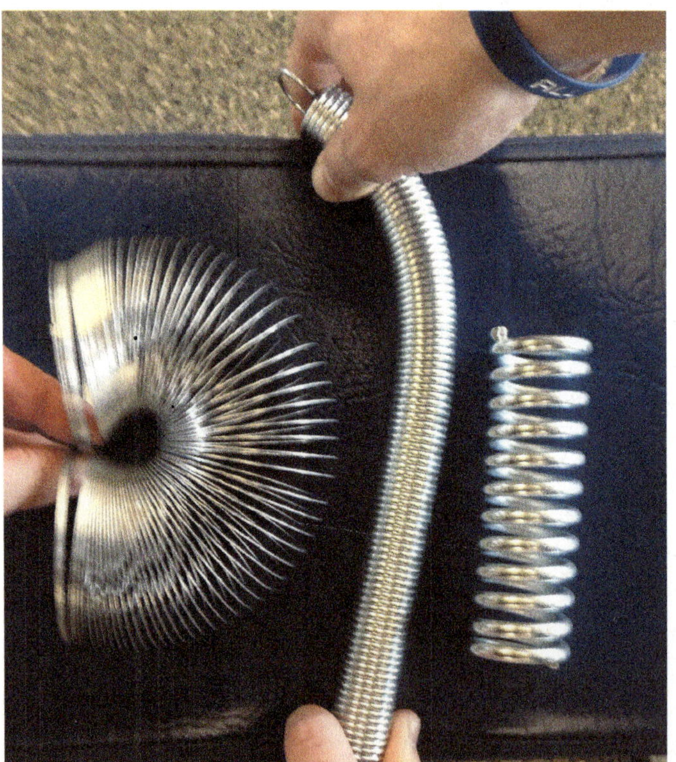

Compliant spring on the left, stiff spring on the right, the middle spring represents both stiffness and compliance.

SECTION 2: Mechanical Efficiency

MECHANICAL EFFICIENCY is an additional consideration for movement. As a coach, I want to increase this variable. Mechanical efficiency is the ratio of external work performed (performance results) to total energy expenditure (work/effort).

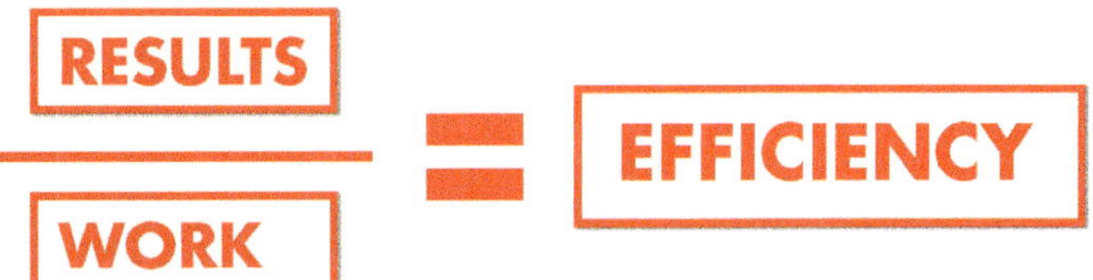

If we can increase the results an athlete can produce while keeping his work the same during competition, then we are creating a more efficient athlete who can perform for longer periods of time. For many sports, it is not about gaining muscle mass, more importantly, it's about increasing efficiency of running, jumping, reacting, bracing, or creating compliant contractions. An efficient/trained athlete utilizes less energy and oxygen during competition when compared to an untrained athlete. We can enhance these increases in the weight room by prescribing exercises that can help increase strength, power, stiffness, and mobility.

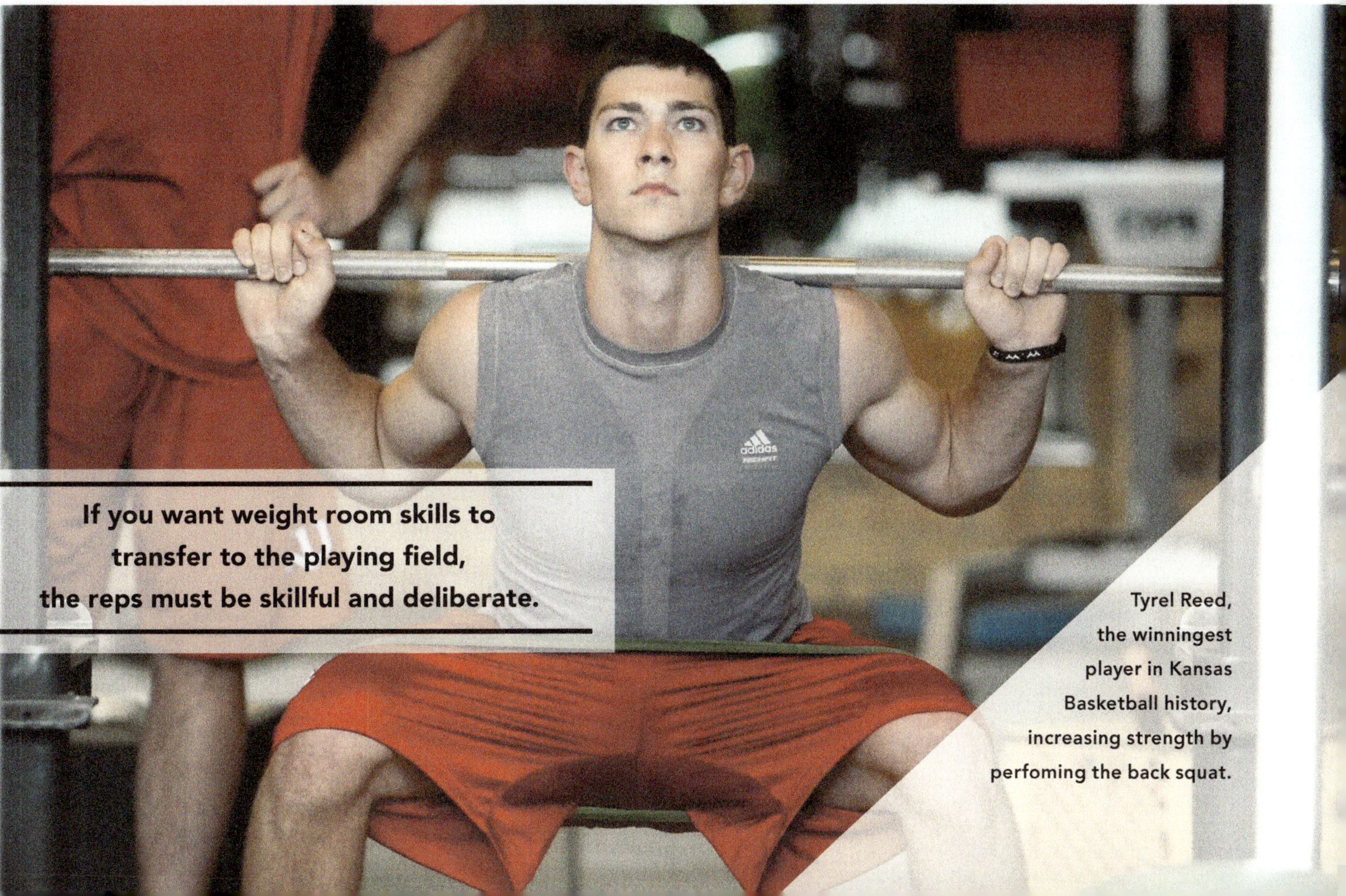

If you want weight room skills to transfer to the playing field, the reps must be skillful and deliberate.

Tyrel Reed, the winningest player in Kansas Basketball history, increasing strength by perfoming the back squat.

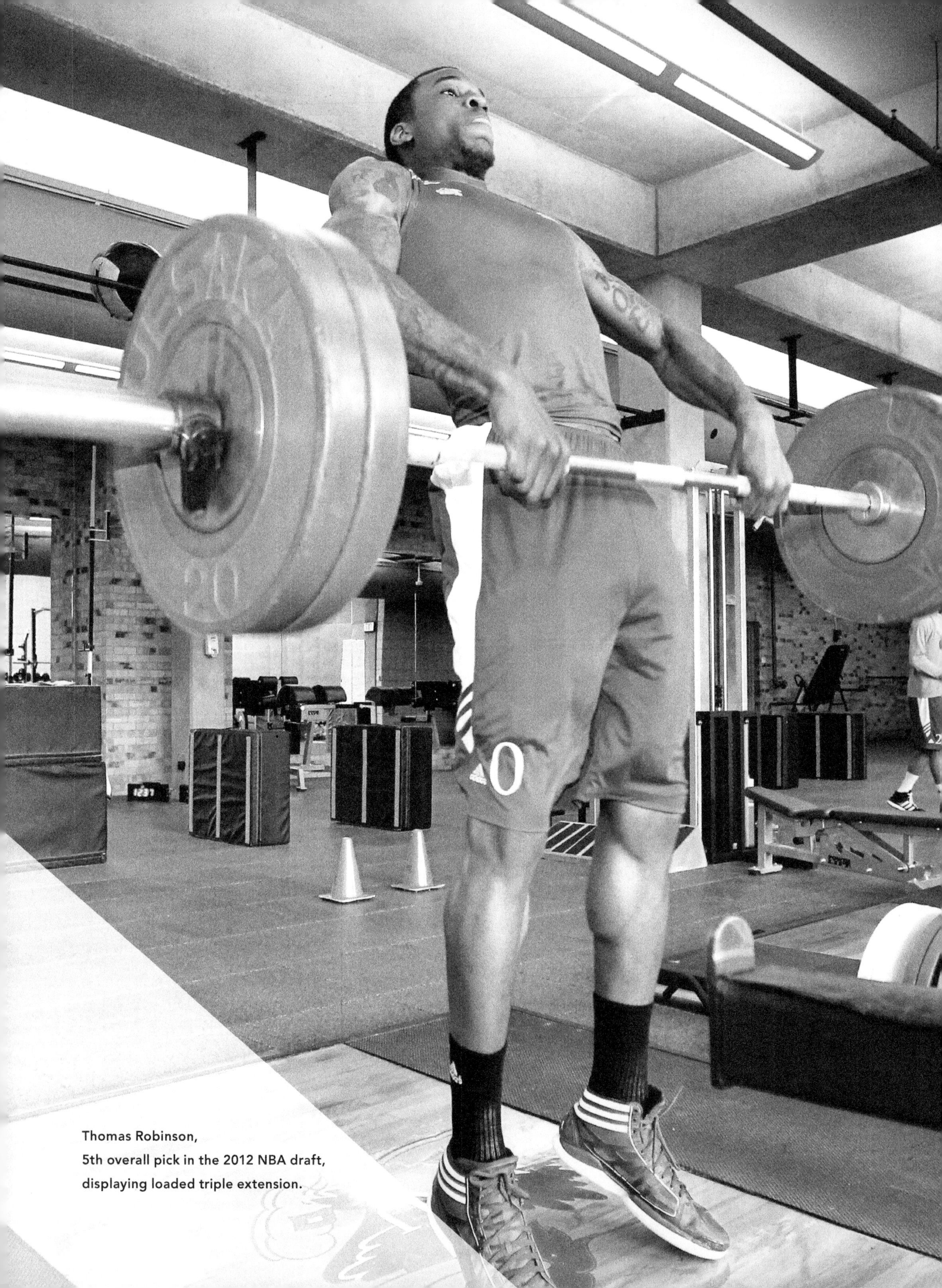

Thomas Robinson,
5th overall pick in the 2012 NBA draft,
displaying loaded triple extension.

BENEFITS OF WEIGHTLIFTING

As a coach, for example, prescribing the exercise, the clean, to an athlete is more than just increasing strength and power. When performed correctly, it encompasses all movement. It is a series of segmented high intensity movements that are coordinated to mimic the ability to create mobility in the joints and muscle stiffness and compliance in the muscles.

At the beginning of the lift, the athlete has to have the mobility to get into a low athletic position. In that position, the athlete must brace the trunk to stabilize and protect the back before he lifts the loaded barbell from the floor. The pull from the floor involves strength in the posterior chain to accelerate through the loaded extension of the ankle, knee, and hip: this is triple extension.

Once the pull is complete, the athlete will receive the bar (catch) on his shoulders. For this to happen, the athlete needs to develop intra abdominal pressure in order to brace against receiving the bar while controlling flexion of the ankle, knee and hip. Controlling flexion of the ankle, knee, and hip while bracing, mimics landing from a jump or landing when running. Once the bar is received, the athlete is in the front squat position. This position requires great ankle mobility, knee stability, hip mobility, lumbar stability, and trunk stiffness to maintain posture. Once stabilized, the athlete is required to stand up. This requires lower body muscle strength and trunk stiffness to accelerate to the standing position. The amount of force that it takes to accelerate a large amount of weight, catch it (brace), and decelerate (or slam on the brakes) is enormous. There is also upper back and arm development that occurs in this lift that are also important.

There are strength and power adaptations that occur throughout the body. The body adapts by building more powerful and stronger muscles, stronger tendons and ligaments, denser bones, and increases proprioceptive awareness for better balance and coordination. If we increase the athletes' strength and power abilities using this loaded skilled movement, then when they run and jump unloaded on the court, field, or track they should become more efficient by increasing strength and power.

The following spread is a frame-by-frame analysis of the clean and how it mimics movement on the basketball court. This analysis can be done for most sports.

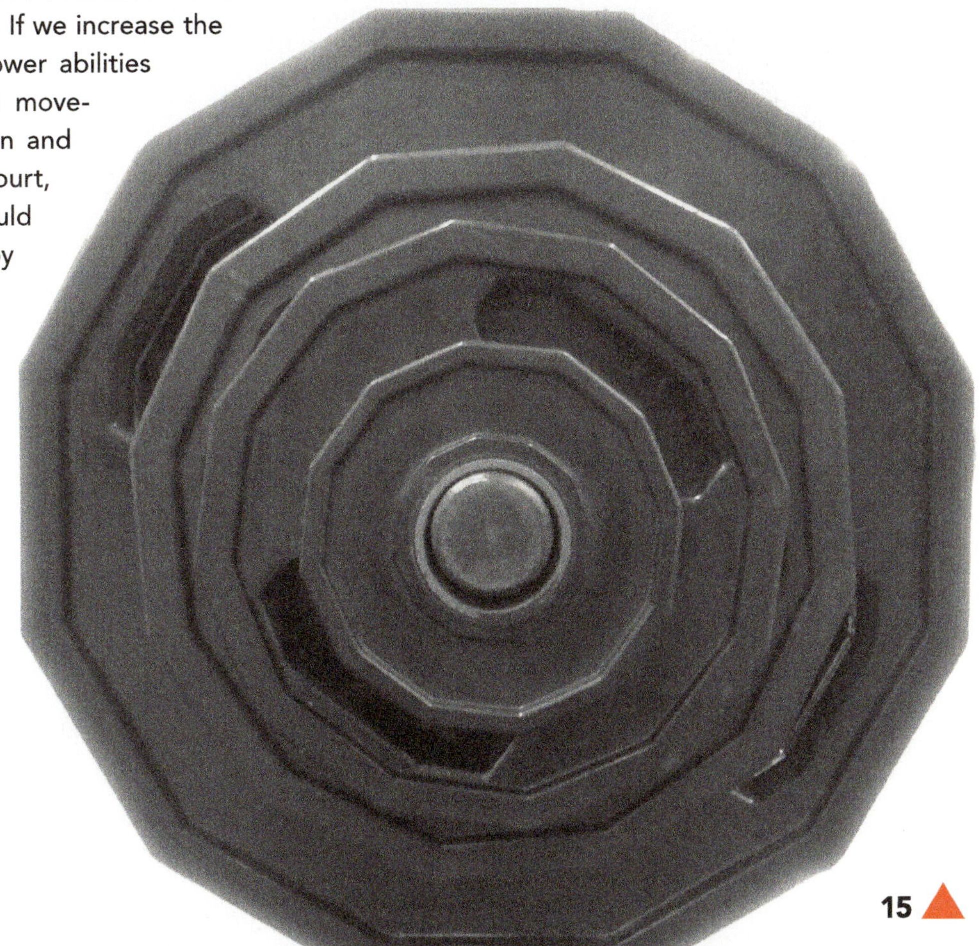

THE CLEAN PROGRESSION:

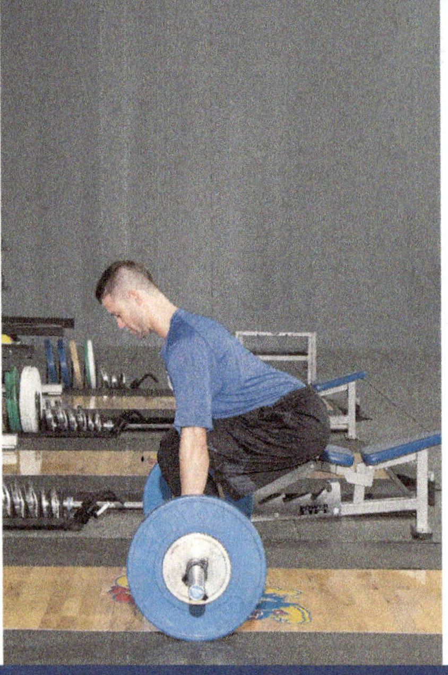

SEATED POSITION

Requires mobility.

Before lifiting one must brace the truck to stabilize and protect the back.

PULL FROM THE FLOOR

While maintaining posture one begins to accelerate the bar from the floor. This requires posterior chain strength.

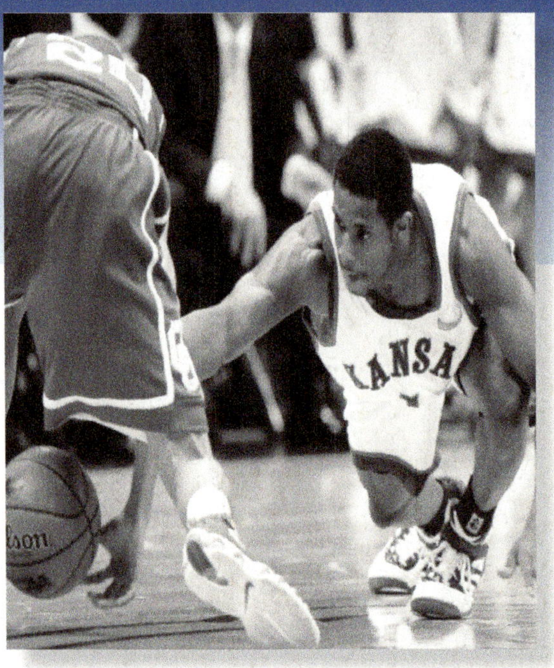

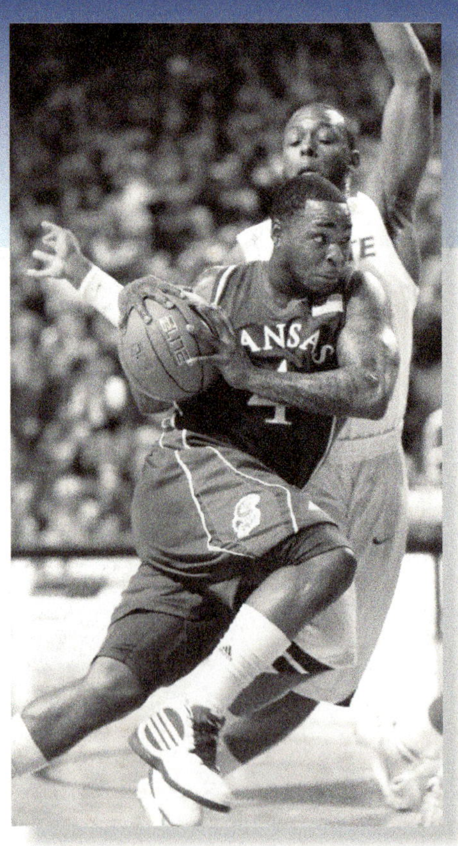

Basketball Movement Specific

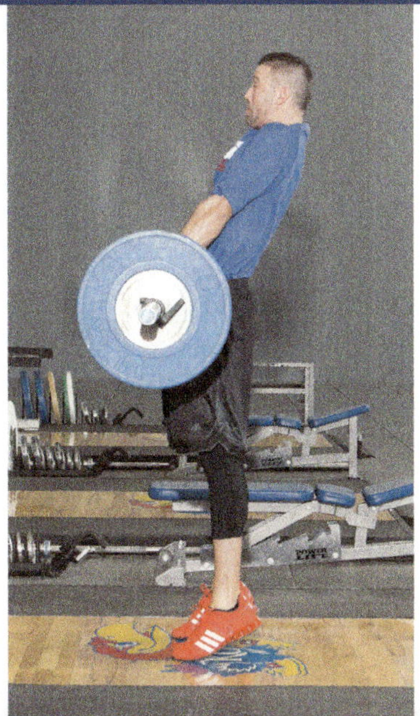

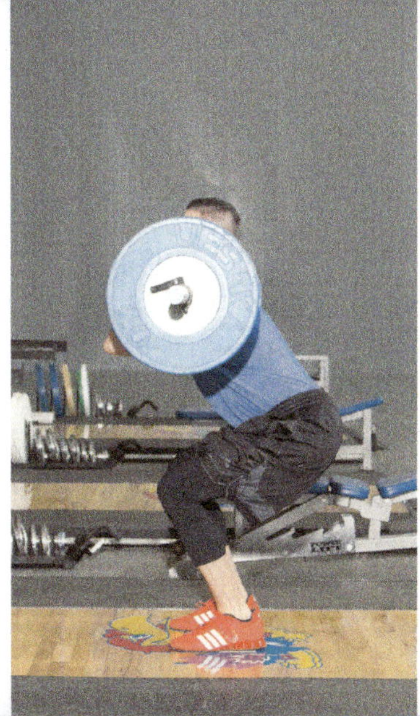

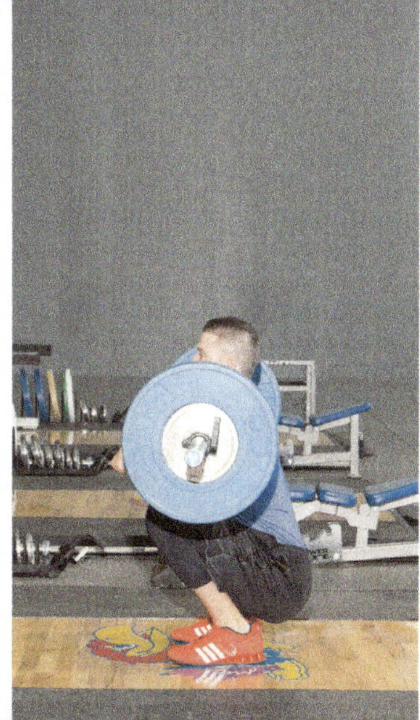

TRIPLE EXTENSION

Loaded through extention.

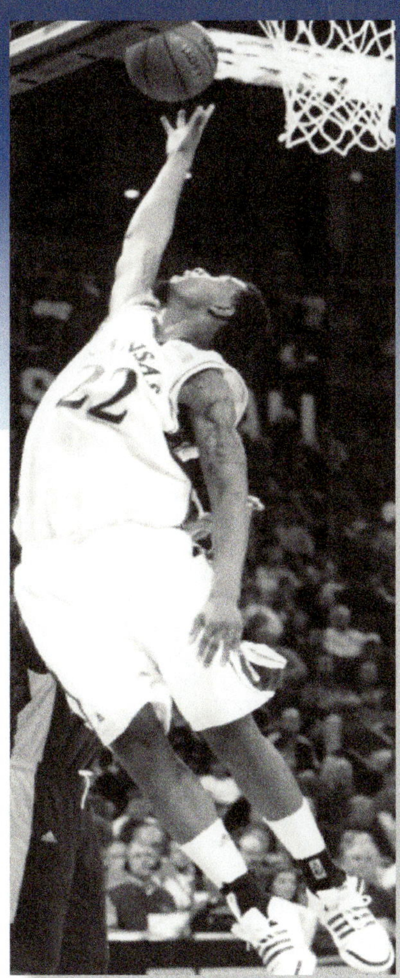

CATCH POSITION

One must create stiffness to control deceleration of the bar (triple flexion).

This mimics landing from a jump or the loading phase while running.

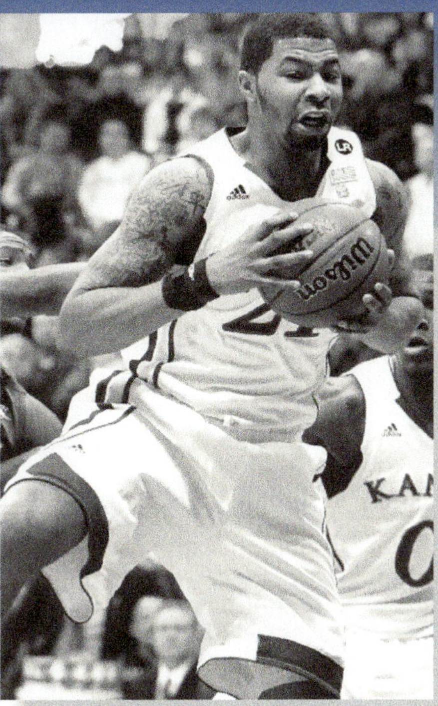

SQUAT

Requires mobility and truck stiffness to maintsin posture.

One must accelerate out of this position. This requires lower body strength.

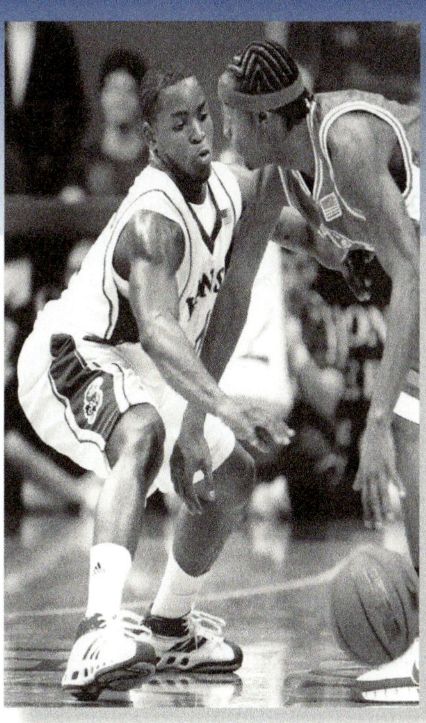

SECTION 3: Lateral Movement

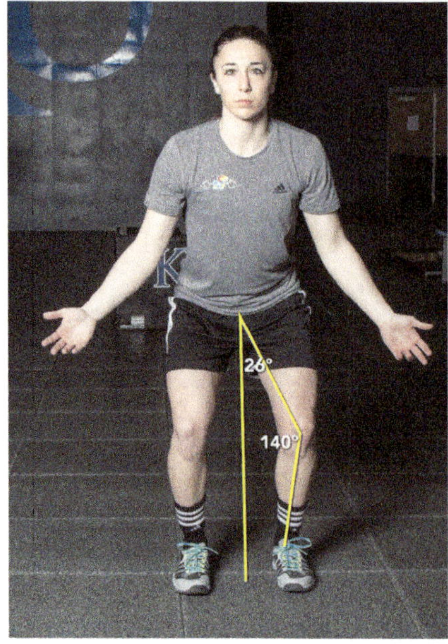

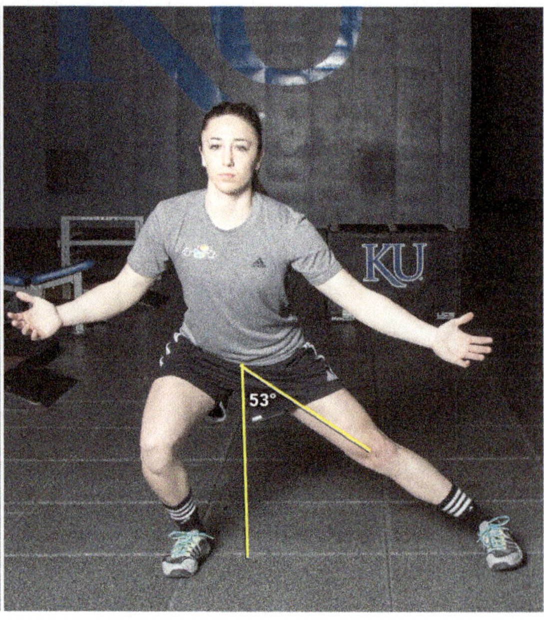

When coaching athletes who play positions that involve lateral movements, one should first examine the movement, the joints, and the ranges of motion involved. If quick lateral agility movements are required for a sports position, the ability to create trunk stiffness is needed. The torso should be rigid in order to move as one unit so it moves easily and efficiently. If a lateral moving athlete carries too much upper body mass or musculature and he is not strong or stiff enough in the torso to create a rigid object when changing direction, then the athlete will not move effectively.

In the first set of pictures the athlete is moving laterally. There is a small range of motion that the athlete moves at the hip. The hip moves approximately twenty-seven degrees in the lateral plane. This is a smaller amount of trainable movement when compared to the vertical plane movements that are illustrated in the next set of pictures.

This side view shows the amount of vertical extension the athlete performs while moving laterally. The summation of ankle, knee, and hip extension is much higher in this plane of movement (106°). Therefore, I believe that I can have a greater training effect using exercises that involve vertical acceleration and deceleration rather than resisted sport-specific lateral training. While resisted lateral movements are effective, our foundation of weightlifting provides the best combination of strength and velocity to increase ground reaction forces to improve agility.

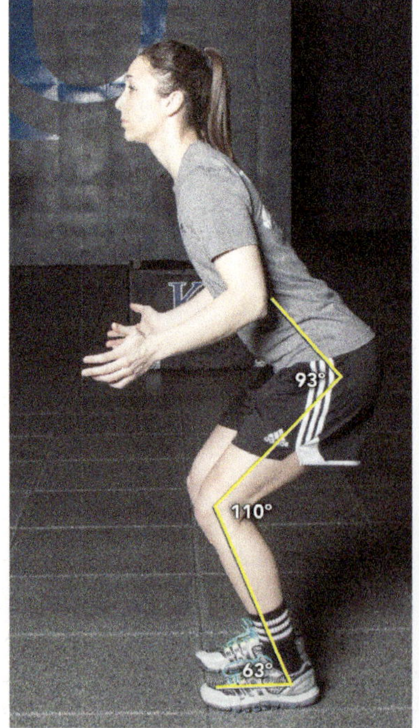

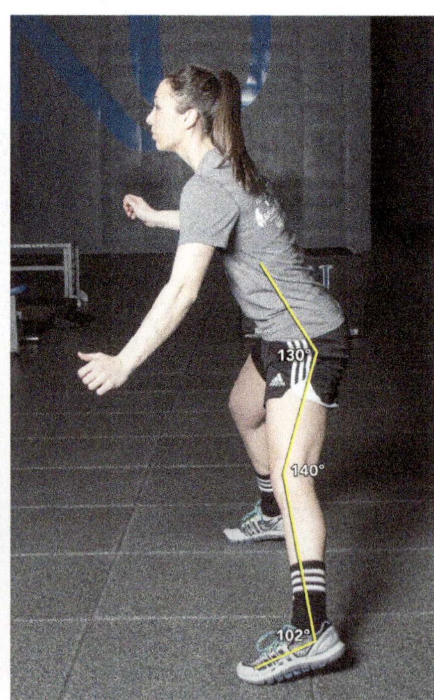

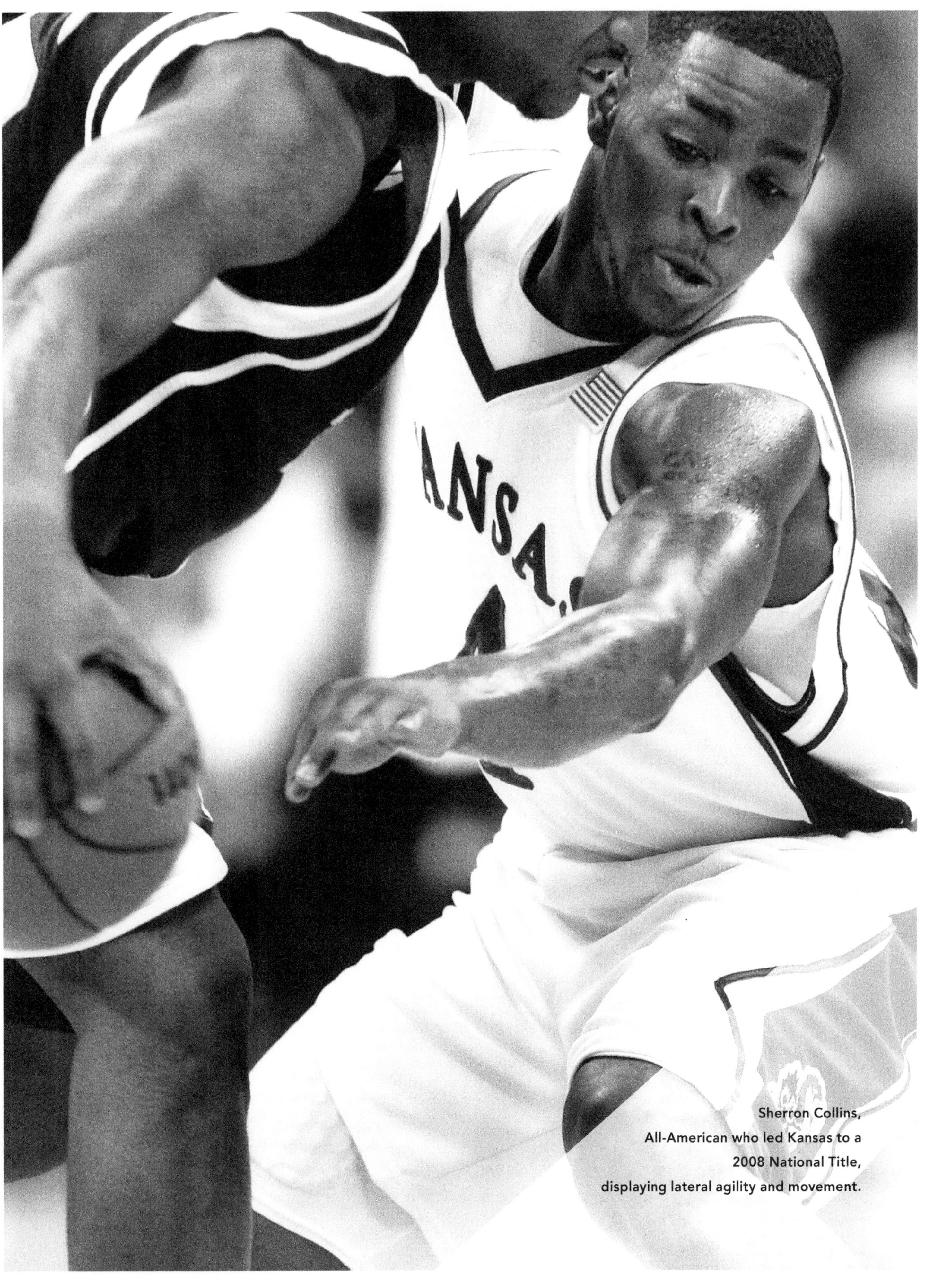

Sherron Collins,
All-American who led Kansas to a
2008 National Title,
displaying lateral agility and movement.

SECTION 4: Assessment

There are numerous standardized and formal tests such as the Functional Movement Screen (FMS), Overhead Squat (OHS) Test or a Titleist Performance Institute (TPI) Assessment. These tests however, are not the only means of assessing all aspects of physical skill. I use the vertical jump test on the force plate with Dr. Wagner at Sparta Science to assess our athlete's movement needs. An athlete could simply take himself through a dynamic warm up and a low intensity lift, and very quickly learn a lot of things about himself:

1. **COORDINATION**
   Are you able to complete basic movements fluidly in a controlled and specific manner?
2. **MOBILITY/MUSCLE IMBALANCES/STRENGTH**
   As you try to complete certain movements ask yourself the following questions:
   1. Does your body compensate by using the wrong muscles to do the work? Perhaps you cannot even get into the correct position.
   2. What does your overhead squat look like?
   3. Do you use one leg more than the other (evidenced by leaning to one side)?
   4. Do you have to excessively lean forward in order to get proper squat depth? This could indicate poor hip mobility and/or poor quad strength, or poor ankle mobility etc.
   5. (1) Do your feet turn out?
      (2) Do your knees cave in?
      (3) Does your pelvis tilt downward (posterior pelvic tilt) as you squat?
   6. Can you hold a solid plank position for a minute and what do your push-ups look like?

After answering the questions, you should have an indication of some areas that might need extra attention in your actual program. It is very important to make sure you are paying attention to your body, learning how you respond to your training as you progress over time. In a sense, you are assessing your body every day during every rep.

Again, we use a simple vertical jump test. It is a standardized counter-movement vertical jump test that is performed six times on the force plate. The reason we use the vertical jump performance test is because it demonstrates the ability to decelerate (load), create stiffness for stability or compliance for mobility (explode), and accelerate (drive), the variables that are correlated to function and performance. How these qualities are sequenced in an athlete's force production into the ground separate them into a lateral, rotational, or linear athlete. Dr. Wagner has statistically proven the importance of proper sequencing regarding athletic abilities. These abilities and how they interact will be discussed in Chapter 2 of the *Power Positions.* Ideally, testing is done once a week so that we can try to control the variables that can affect performance: Nutrition, stress, sleep needs, fatigue, soreness, injury, etc.

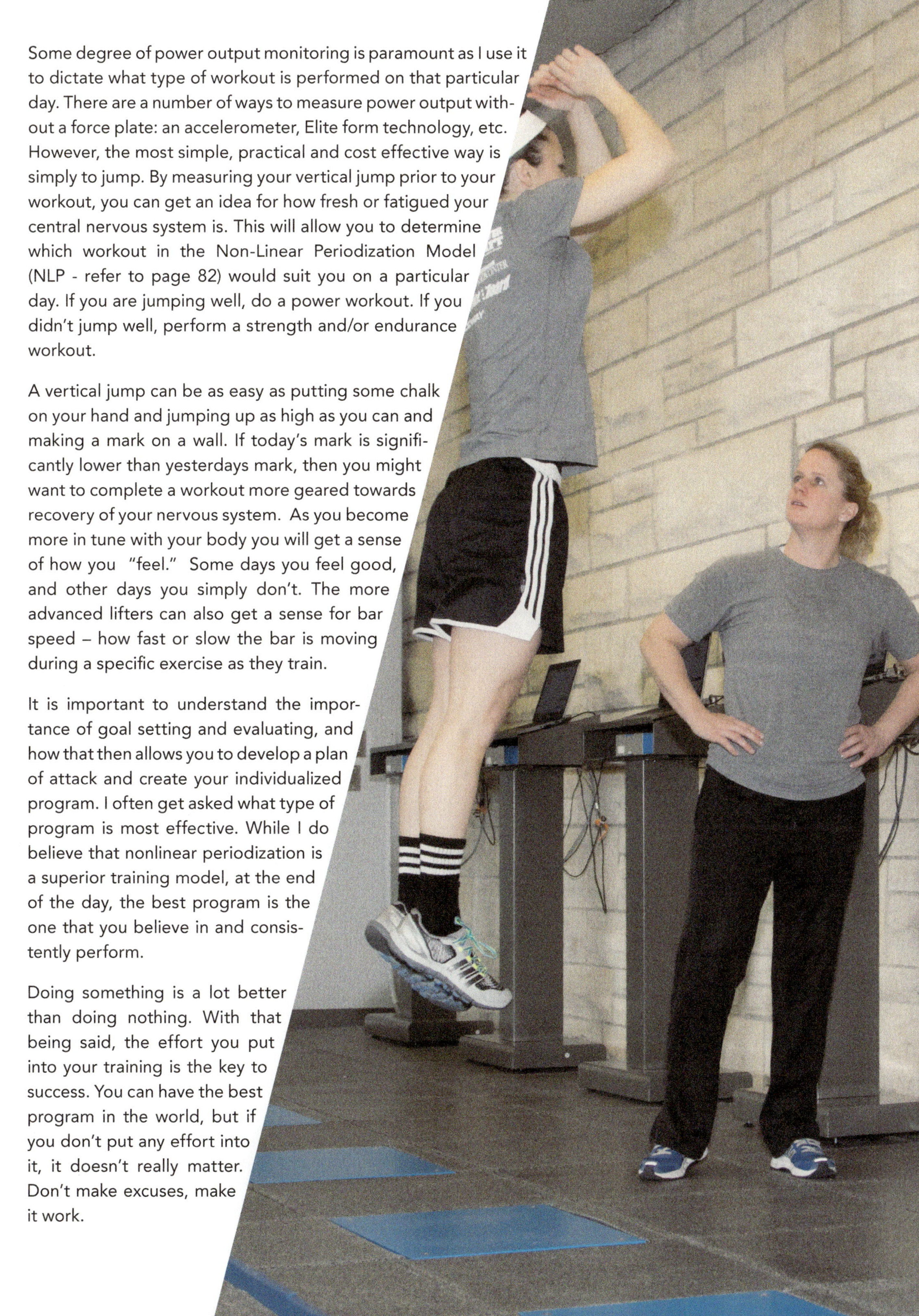

Some degree of power output monitoring is paramount as I use it to dictate what type of workout is performed on that particular day. There are a number of ways to measure power output without a force plate: an accelerometer, Elite form technology, etc. However, the most simple, practical and cost effective way is simply to jump. By measuring your vertical jump prior to your workout, you can get an idea for how fresh or fatigued your central nervous system is. This will allow you to determine which workout in the Non-Linear Periodization Model (NLP - refer to page 82) would suit you on a particular day. If you are jumping well, do a power workout. If you didn't jump well, perform a strength and/or endurance workout.

A vertical jump can be as easy as putting some chalk on your hand and jumping up as high as you can and making a mark on a wall. If today's mark is significantly lower than yesterdays mark, then you might want to complete a workout more geared towards recovery of your nervous system. As you become more in tune with your body you will get a sense of how you "feel." Some days you feel good, and other days you simply don't. The more advanced lifters can also get a sense for bar speed – how fast or slow the bar is moving during a specific exercise as they train.

It is important to understand the importance of goal setting and evaluating, and how that then allows you to develop a plan of attack and create your individualized program. I often get asked what type of program is most effective. While I do believe that nonlinear periodization is a superior training model, at the end of the day, the best program is the one that you believe in and consistently perform.

Doing something is a lot better than doing nothing. With that being said, the effort you put into your training is the key to success. You can have the best program in the world, but if you don't put any effort into it, it doesn't really matter. Don't make excuses, make it work.

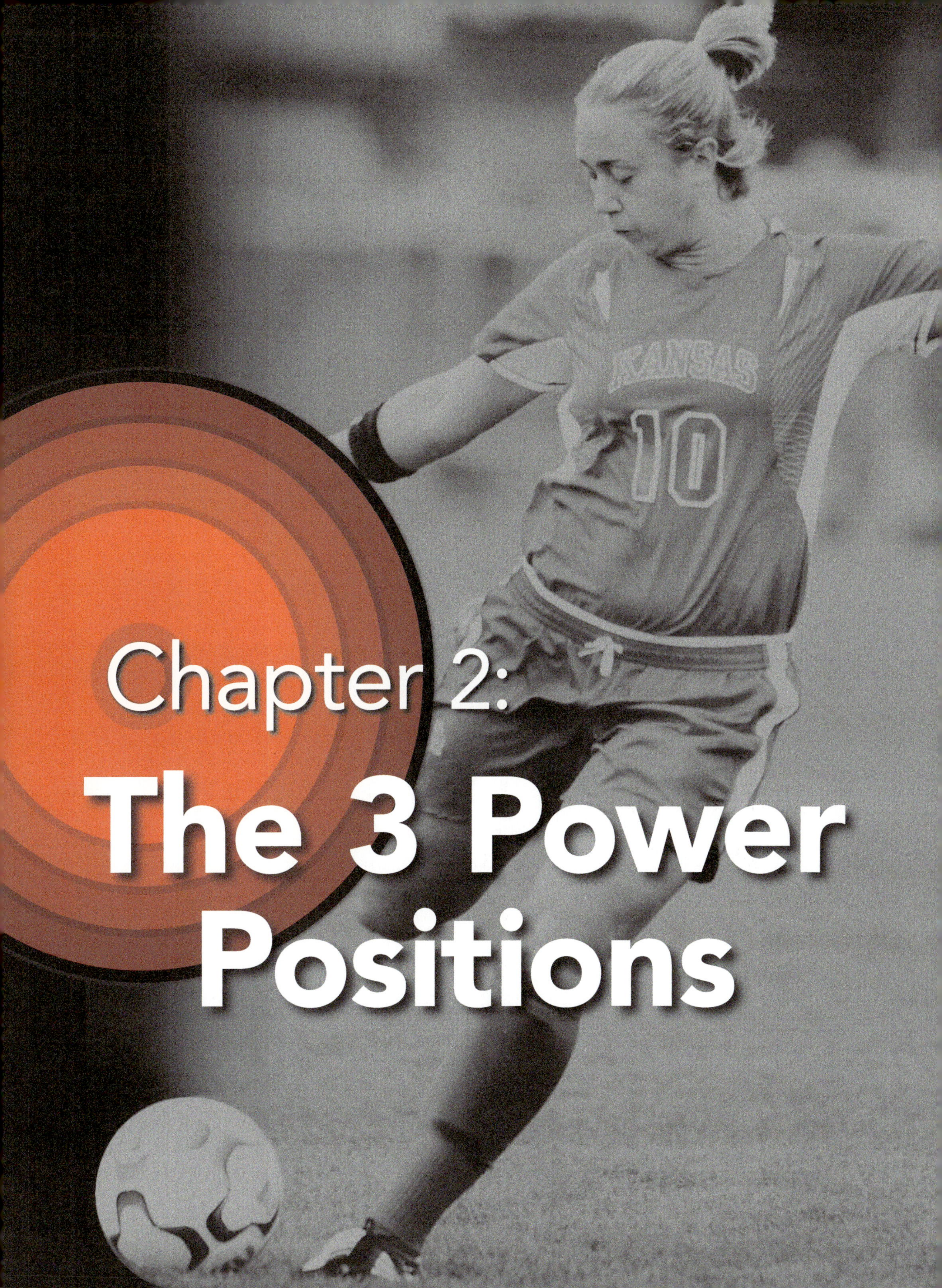

Chapter 2: The 3 Power Positions

SECTION 1: Training is not about the sport, training is about the position.

You now have a basic understanding of human movement. The next step is learning the specific attributes that separate each of the 3 Power Positions.

The amount of stiffness and/or compliance an athlete can create has a link to athletic performance. For example, have you ever seen an athlete jumping in place or performing tuck jumps before a game or event? This athlete is trying use short, fast, ballistic muscle movements to increase stiffness because, instinctively, he may feel too loose or compliant to perform his skill efficiently.

On the other hand, have you ever seen an athlete stretching, performing torso rotations, or swinging their arms before a game or before he gets in the blocks for a race? This athlete is trying to decrease stiffness or increase compliance with long healthy muscular movements because he may feel too stiff or 'too tight' to perform his skill for competition. Too much stiffness can have a negative effect on performance. What the athlete is doing before performing a skill speaks volumes to me. Do they feel too loose (compliant) or are they too tight (stiff) for the skill they are performing?

The following chapter will explain the importance of stiffness and compliance as it relates to specific sports positions and times of the year. It's not the sport you play, it is the position you play. The following are the three power positions and programs needed to excel at every sport position.

1. Lateral-Reactive – **Do you primarily play defense, jump, move laterally, or react to someone or something?**

These are examples but are not limited to the following:

- Basketball player
- Defensive back in American football
- Inside receiver in American football
- Linebacker
- Running back
- Defensive end in American football
- Setter in volleyball
- Jumper in track and field
- Middle blocker in volleyball
- Defensive back in soccer
- Shortstop in baseball or softball
- Offensive lineman in American football

2. Rotational - Is rotation a primary movement in your sport?

These are examples of athletes who produce rotational power:

- Tennis player
- Baseball pitcher
- Softball pitcher
- Ice Hockey athlete
- Golfer
- In-the pocket quarterback in American football
- Outside hitter in volleyball (also linear)
- Discus Thrower
- Javelin Thrower

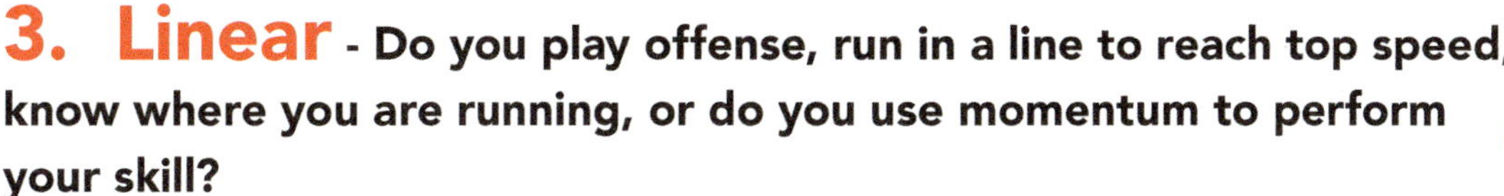

3. Linear - Do you play offense, run in a line to reach top speed, know where you are running, or do you use momentum to perform your skill?

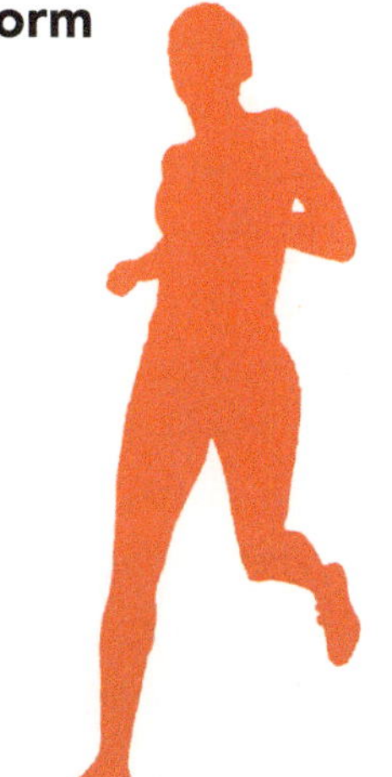

These are examples but are not limited to the following:

For Speed

- Safety in American football
- Outside receiver in American football
- Track sprinter/middle distance
- Forward in soccer
- Outfielder in baseball or softball
- Defensive Lineman in American football
- Outside hitter in volleyball (also rotational)

Do you become so efficient in your sport that you require mobility exercises to stay healthy? These are examples of athletes who need to increase muscle compliance to increase mobility due to increased stiffness

For Mobility

- Triathlete
- Swimmer
- Long distance runner
- Cyclist

Each program has specific goals because different sport positions require different sequencing in the force production from the ground up through the body. **Therefore, training is not just about the sport, training is the about the position.**

Inthefollowingsectionsthepositionswillbeemphasizedbythefollowingcolors:

BLUE - lateral reactive, GREEN - rotational , RED - linear.

SECTION 2: Defining the Lateral Athlete

Have you ever watched a high-level basketball player move on the court? Most of the braking movements for the lateral athlete occur through contact on the ground via the mobile ankle and stable knee. This lateral or reactive athlete is constantly braking to change direction to accelerate vertically, laterally or horizontally. The healthy lateral athlete uses a moderate amount of load or deceleration capabilities but has a great ability to create stiffness to explode and accelerate. This athlete rarely runs in a straight line therefore they have a low amount of drive.

Many of the ground reaction forces are absorbed and utilized by the ankle and knee joints. The ankle must be trained to be mobile through a strong compliant calf. The knee must be trained to be stable through a strong quadriceps group. In order to be efficient at changing direction, the athlete needs to keep his torso rigid (stiff/strong) to stay erect. There is no time to waste by bending over at the hip or the torso to absorb force when you have to react. Many coaches call this core strength. This is one of the reasons that too much muscle mass in the upper body can actually have a negative effect on performance. If the athlete is muscle bound in the upper body and he has to quickly change direction, the increased amount of mass may slow the athlete down because it will require more strength to change direction or stop the momentum of the athlete's upper body.

TRAINING MISCONCEPTIONS ABOUT THE LATERAL ATHLETE

To ask a basketball player, defensive back, or jumper, who is anterior chain (ankle-calf and knee-quadriceps) dominant to perform track sprints at top speed would put the lateral or reactive athlete at a disadvantage. Track sprinters who reach and maintain top speed are posterior chain (ankle-calf, knee-hamstring, and hip-glutes) dominant because they run in a predetermined path. The lateral or reactive athlete attempting a posterior chain dominant workout or event will have an increased chance of injury, such as a strained hamstring, because he is not primarily trained to perform posterior chain dominant activities at top speed. Most lateral or reactive athletes should have an anterior chain dominant quality that puts them at an advantage to brake before acceleration. This is what makes them highly reactive athlete.

For example, if/when a basketball player is trained on the track by doing sprints to top speed in the pre-season and then asked to be reactive on the court when in-season practice begins, the athlete is at a disadvantage to perform quick and reactive skills. He hasn't trained his anterior chain properly to stop. Since the athlete hasn't been trained to decelerate or stop, there is an increased risk of injury (possible ligament sprain/tear) because the training wasn't specific to the movements that occur on the court. He has been accelerating and running a straight line on the track instead of performing agility or plyometric drills. This is not specific training, and demonstrates the importance of specificity of training.

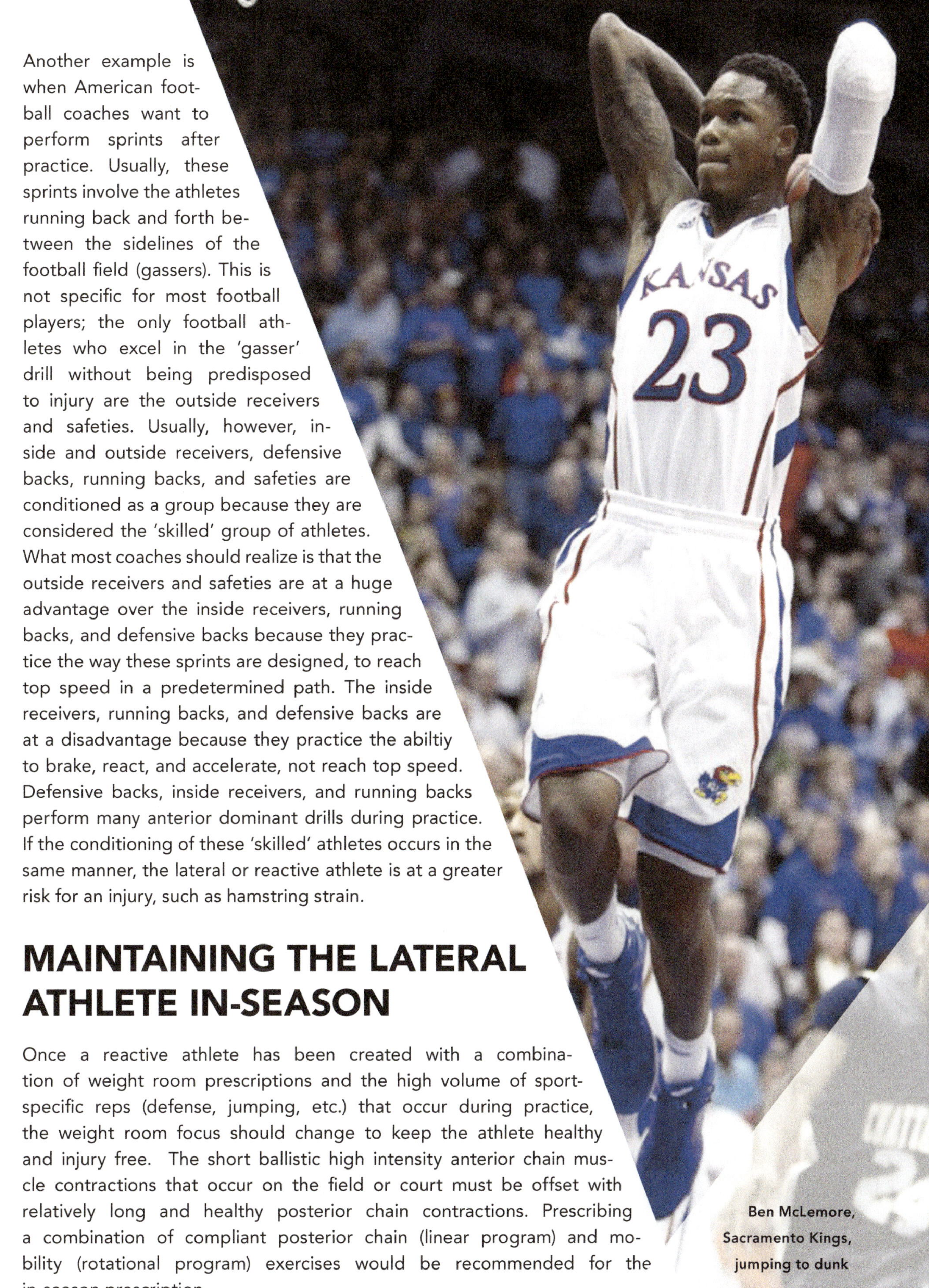

Another example is when American football coaches want to perform sprints after practice. Usually, these sprints involve the athletes running back and forth between the sidelines of the football field (gassers). This is not specific for most football players; the only football athletes who excel in the 'gasser' drill without being predisposed to injury are the outside receivers and safeties. Usually, however, inside and outside receivers, defensive backs, running backs, and safeties are conditioned as a group because they are considered the 'skilled' group of athletes. What most coaches should realize is that the outside receivers and safeties are at a huge advantage over the inside receivers, running backs, and defensive backs because they practice the way these sprints are designed, to reach top speed in a predetermined path. The inside receivers, running backs, and defensive backs are at a disadvantage because they practice the abiltiy to brake, react, and accelerate, not reach top speed. Defensive backs, inside receivers, and running backs perform many anterior dominant drills during practice. If the conditioning of these 'skilled' athletes occurs in the same manner, the lateral or reactive athlete is at a greater risk for an injury, such as hamstring strain.

MAINTAINING THE LATERAL ATHLETE IN-SEASON

Once a reactive athlete has been created with a combination of weight room prescriptions and the high volume of sport-specific reps (defense, jumping, etc.) that occur during practice, the weight room focus should change to keep the athlete healthy and injury free. The short ballistic high intensity anterior chain muscle contractions that occur on the field or court must be offset with relatively long and healthy posterior chain contractions. Prescribing a combination of compliant posterior chain (linear program) and mobility (rotational program) exercises would be recommended for the in-season prescription.

Ben McLemore, Sacramento Kings, jumping to dunk

Year Round Training Concepts for the Lateral Athlete

When to Perform	Off Season	Pre Season	In Season	Post Season
Which Program	Lateral	Lateral	Rotational or Linear	Rotational or Linear
Purpose	Increase total power and anterior chain strength	Increase total power and anterior chain strength	Increase total power and posterior chain strength	Increase total power and posterior chain strength
	CREATE STIFFNESS		**MAINTAIN COMPLIANCE**	
Movements	1° Short ballistic movements to increase ability to create muscular stiffness 2° Bracing and posturing exercises 3° Long healthy movements to increase muscle compliance and joint mobility	1° Short ballistic movements to increase ability to create muscular stiffness 2° Bracing and posturing exercises 3° Long healthy movements to increase muscle compliance and joint mobility	1° Long healthy contractions to increase joint mobility and muscular compliance to counteract ballistic movements in sport competition and practice 2° Low intensity rotational movements and complete ranges of motion	1° Long healthy contractions to increase joint mobility and muscular compliance to counteract ballistic movements in sport competition and practice 2° Low intensity rotational movements and complete ranges of motion
Emphasis	1° Strength (load- based resistance training) 2° Power (velocity-based resistance training)	1° Strength (load- based resistance training) 2° Power (velocity-based resistance training)	1° Power (velocity-based resistance training) 2° Strength (load- based resistance training)	1° Power (velocity-based resistance training) 2° Strength (load-based resistance training)

Movement skills to create the Lateral Athlete in the off-season and pre-season

(see movement skills in Section 5)

Position	Off season and pre season needs	Emphasis Quick Response	Development	Movement	Action
Lateral	1° Anterior Chain Development 2° Posterior Chain Development	1° Depth jump landing mechanics 2° Depth Jumps 3° Short response plyometrics 4° Agility 5° Speed Development 6° Long response plyometrics	1° Stiffness 2° Compliance	1° Reactive 2° Predetermined	1° Braking 2° Accelerating

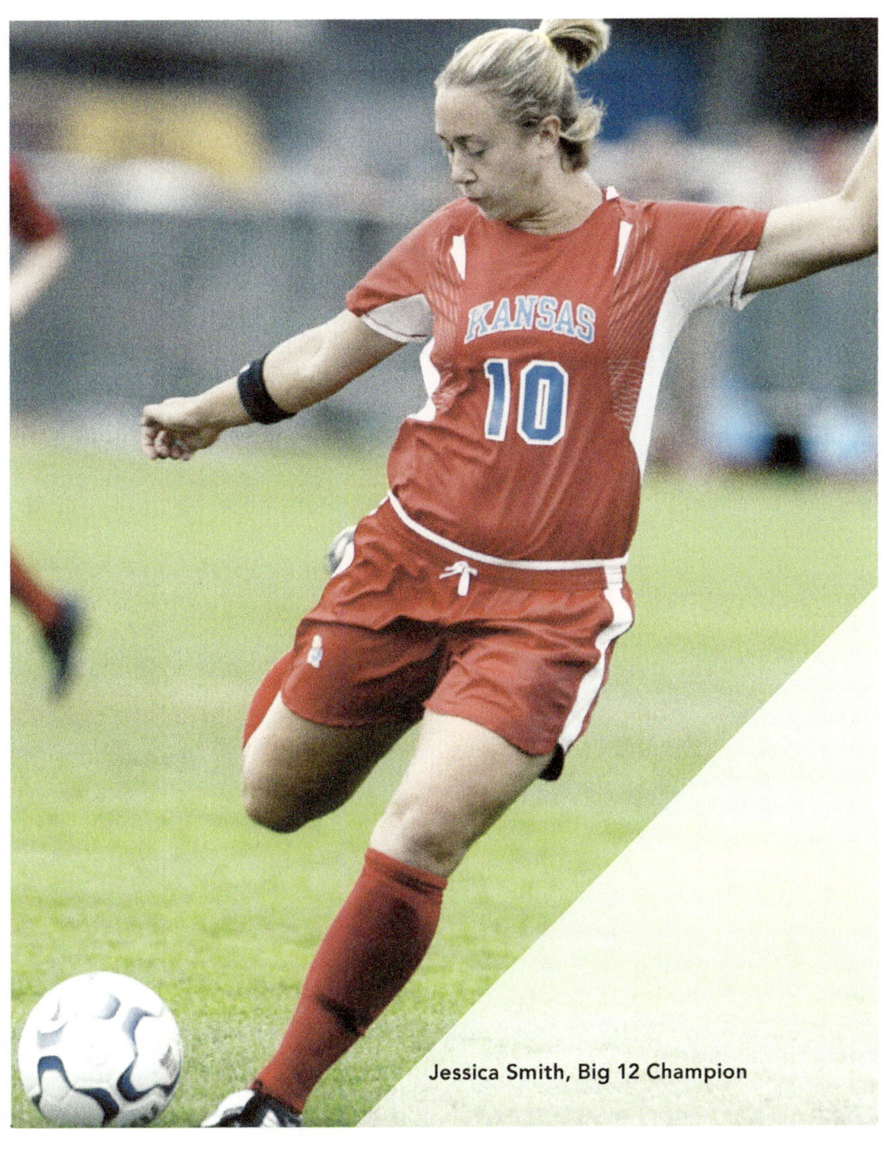

Jessica Smith, Big 12 Champion

THE WORKOUTS: the Lateral-Reactive Athlete

The following is a simple calendar that represents what a training month can look like.

ATHLETE
SAMPLE MONTHLY CALENDAR

SUNDAY	MONDAY	TUESDAY	WEDNESDAY	THURSDAY	FRIDAY	SATURDAY
	DAY 1	*MOVEMENT SKILLS*	**DAY 2**	*MOVEMENT SKILLS*	**DAY 3**	
	DAY 1	*MOVEMENT SKILLS*	**DAY 2**	*MOVEMENT SKILLS*	**DAY 3**	
	DAY 1	*MOVEMENT SKILLS*	**DAY 2**	*MOVEMENT SKILLS*	**DAY 3**	
	DAY 1	*MOVEMENT SKILLS*	**DAY 2**	*MOVEMENT SKILLS*	**DAY 3**	
	DAY 1	*MOVEMENT SKILLS*	**DAY 2**	*MOVEMENT SKILLS*	**DAY 3**	

The following page's contain workouts for the beginner, intermediate, advanced and elite lateral-reactive athlete.

Eight Week Movement Plan for the Lateral-Reactive Athlete

(see movement skills in Section 5)

	Week 1	Week 2	Week 3	Week 4	Week 5	Week 6	Week 7	Week 8
Box Height (if applicable)	**12 inches**	**14 inches**	**16 inches**	**18 inches**	**22 inches**	**24 inches**	**28 inches**	**30 inches**
Landing Mechanics-Depth Jumps								
Sets x Reps	2 x 5	2 x 5	2 x 5	1 x 3				
Depth Jumps								
Sets x Reps	1 x 5	1 x 5	1 x 3	4 x 2	4 x 3	4 x 3	4 x 3	4 x 3
Short Response Plyometrics								
6 inches								
Linear (Foot Contacts)	100	140	180	200				
Lateral (Foot Contacts)	24	32	40	50				
12 inches								
Linear (Foot Contacts)					100	140	180	200
Lateral (Foot Contacts)					24	32	40	50
Agility Drills (Total Reps)								
Acceleration	10	12	15	17	20	22	25	27
Deceleration	10	12	15	17	20	22	25	27
Speed Development (Sets)	1 set	1 set	1 set	1 set	2 sets	2 sets	2 sets	2 sets

LATERAL-REACTIVE BEGINNER

Day 1	Hypertrophy		
Exercise	**Sets**	**Reps**	**Purpose**
A1) Goblet Squat	3	10	Lower Body Anterior Chain
A2) Front Plank	3	30 s	Stiffness
B1) Bodyweight Squat	3	10	Lower Body Posterior Chain
B2) Side Plank L/R	3	30 s	Stiffness
B3) Pushup (Use Incline if Needed)	3	10	Upper Body Horizontal Push
C1) Bodyweight Reverse Lunge	3	5/5	Lower Body Anterior Chain
C2) Farmer's Walk	3	20 yds	Stiffness
C3) Inverted Row (Use Incline if Needed)	3	10	Upper Body Horizontal Pull

Day 2	Power		
Exercise	**Sets**	**Reps**	**Purpose**
A1) Jump Rope	3	30 s	Lower Body Anterior Chain
A2) Bodyweight Split Jump	3	3/3	Total Body Explosive
B1) 2 Leg Depth Jump (Landing Mechanics)	3	5	Lower Body Anterior Chain/Stiffness
B2) Lat Pulldown	3	6	Upper Body Vertical Pull
C1) Ice Skater Jump	3	5/5	Total Body Lateral Explosive
C2) 1 Arm Farmer's Walk	3	20 yds	Stiffness
D1) DB Squat	3	5	Lower Body Posterior Chain
D2) DB Incline Bench Press	3	5	Upper Body Vertical Push

Day 3	Strength		
Exercise	**Sets**	**Reps**	**Purpose**
A1) 1 Leg Squat	3	5/5	Lower Body Anterior Chain
A2) Plate Torso Twist	3	6/6	Compliance
A3) Leg Lowers	3	8	Stiffness
B1) Reverse Lunge	3	6/6	Lower Body Anterior Chain
B2) DB Lateral Bend	3	8/8	Lateral Movement
B3) Bench	3	8	Upper Body Horizontal Push
C1) Leg Extension	3	8	Lower Body Anterior Chain
C2) Seated Row	3	8	Upper Body Horizontal Pull
C3) Lateral Windmill	3	10/10	Lateral Movement

LATERAL-REACTIVE INTERMEDIATE

Day 1 — Hypertrophy

Exercise	Sets	Reps	Purpose
A1) 1 Leg Squat	4	8/8	Lower Body Anterior Chain
A2) 1 Arm DB OH Press	4	10/10	Upper Body Vertical Push/Stiffness
B1) Reverse Lunge	4	8/8	Lower Body Anterior Chain
B2) Hanging Knee Raise	4	10	Stiffness
B3) Seated Row	4	10	Upper Body Horizontal Pull
C1) Front Squat	4	6	Lower Body Anterior Chain
C2) 1 Arm DB Farmer's Walk	4	20 yds	Stiffness
C3) Lateral Windmill	4	10/10	Lateral Movement

Day 2 — Power

Exercise	Sets	Reps	Purpose
A1) Jump Rope	4	30s	Lower Body Anterior Chain
A2) Squat Jump	4	5	Total Body Explosive
A3) DB Side Bend	4	6/6	Stiffness
B1) Split Jump	4	3/3	Total Body Explosive/Anterior Chain
B2) DB Incline Bench Press	4	6	Upper Body Vertical Push
B3) Plate Torso Twist	4	6/6	Stiffness
C1) Box Jump	4	4	Total Body Explosive
C2) 2 Leg Depth Jump	4	5	Lower Body Anterior Chain/Stiffness
C3) Pull Up	4	5	Upper Body Vertical Pull

Day 3 — Strength

Exercise	Sets	Reps	Purpose
A1) Goblet Squat	4	8	Lower Body Anterior Chain
A2) Side Plank L/R	4	30 s	Stiffness
A3) Bench Press	4	8	Upper Body Horizontal Push
B1) Deadlift	4	6	Lower Body Posterior Chain
B2) Ice Skater Jump	4	6/6	Lateral Movement/Stiffness
B3) 1 Arm DB Row	4	8/8	Upper Body Horizontal Pull
C1) Reverse Lunge	4	5/5	Lower Body Anterior Chain
C2) PVC Behind the Neck Press	4	8	Upper Body Veritcal Push/ Mobility
C3) Figure 4 Stretch	4	30 s	Compliance

LATERAL-REACTIVE ADVANCED

Day 1	Speed - Strength		
Exercise	**Sets**	**Reps**	**Purpose**
A1) Jump Squat	4	5	Total Body Explosive
A2) 1 Arm DB Row	4	8/8	Upper Body Horizontal Pull
A3) Side Plank L/R	4	30 s	Stiffness
B1) Clean Drop Squat	4	4	Total Body/Mobility
B2) DB Incline Bench Press	4	8	Upper Body Vertical Push
B3) 1-Arm Farmer's Walk	4	20 yds	Stiffness
C1) Hang Power Snatch	4	3	Total Body Explosive
C2) Pull Up	4	5	Upper Body Vertical Pull
C3) 1-Leg Squat	4	3/3	Lower Body Anterior Chain

Day 2	Strength - Speed		
Exercise	**Sets**	**Reps**	**Purpose**
A1) Heel Elevated OH Squat	4	5	Lower Body Anterior Chain/Mobility
A2) Side Bend	4	6/6	Stiffness
A3) Jump Rope	4	30s	Lower Body Anterior Chain
B1) Hang Clean - Front Squat	4	3	Total Body Explosive
B2) Plyo Pull Up	4	5	Upper Body Vertical Pull /Stiffness /Anterior Chain
B3) Side Hip Lift	4	8/8	Stiffness
C1) Power Jerk	4	2	Upper Body Vertical Push
C2) Leg Extension	4	5/5	Lower Body Anterior Chain
C3) Farmer's Walk	4	20 yds	Stiffness

Day 3	Strength		
Exercise	**Sets**	**Reps**	**Purpose**
A1) OH Drop Squat	4	6	Lower Body Anterior Chain/Mobility
A2) 1 Arm DB OH Press	4	8/8	Upper Body Vertical Push/Stiffness
B1) Front Squat	4	6	Lower Body Anterior Chain
B2) Calf Raise	4	8	Posterior Chain
B3) Inverted Row	4	8	Upper Body Horizontal Pull
C1) Hang Power Clean	4	4	Total Body Explosive
C2) Lateral Windmill	4	8/8	Lateral Movement
C3) 1 Leg Glute Bridge	4	8/8	Lower Body Posterior Chain

LATERAL-REACTIVE ELITE

Day 1 — Speed - Strength

Exercise	Sets	Reps	Purpose
A1) Clean Drop Squat	4	5	Total Body/Mobility
A2) Plyo Rotational Pull Up	4	4/4	Upper Body Vertical Pull/Stiffness /Anterior Chain
A3) Hanging Knee Raise	4	10	Stiffness
B1) Hang Power Snatch	4	4	Total Body Explosive
B2) Plyo Pushup	4	8	Upper Body Horizontal Push/Explosive
B3) 1 Arm Bulgarian Split Squat	4	5/5	Lower Body Posterior Chain/Mobility /Stiffness
C1) Hang Clean - Front Squat	4	3	Total Body Explosive
C2) Ice Skater Jump	4	5/5	Total Body Lateral Explosive
C3) BB 1 Leg Squat	4	3/3	Lower Body Anterior Chain/Stiffness

Day 2 — Strength - Speed

Exercise	Sets	Reps	Purpose
A1) OH Drop Squat	4	5	Lower Body Anterior Chain/Mobility
A2) Lateral Windmill	4	6/6	Lateral Movement
A3) Seated Row	4	8	Upper Body Horizontal Pull
B1) Split Jerk	4	2/2	Total Body Explosive/Vertical Push
B2) MB OH Slam	4	6	Total Body Explosive
B3) 1 Leg Box Jump	4	4/4	Total Body Explosive/Stiffness
C1) Hang Power Clean	4	2	Total Body Explosive
C2) 2 Leg Depth Jump (Landing Mechanics)	4	5	Lower Body Anterior Chain/Stiffness
C3) 1 Arm OH Farmer's Walk	4	20 yds	Stiffness

Day 3 — Strength

Exercise	Sets	Reps	Purpose
A1) BB Split Squat	4	5/5	Lower Body Posterior Chain
A2) 1 Arm DB Hang Power Snatch	4	4/4	Total Body Explosive/Stiffness
B1) Incline Bench Press	4	6	Upper Body Vertical Push
B2) Wide Grip Pull Up	4	6	Upper Body Vertical Pull/Stiffness
B3) 1 Arm Farmer's Walk	4	20 yds	Stiffness
C1) Front Squat	4	6	Lower Body Anterior Chain
C2) DB Lateral Squat	4	5/5	Lower Body Posterior Chain/Mobility
C3) Plate Lateral Bend	4	6/6	Stiffness

SECTION 3: Defining the Rotational Athlete

Have you ever watched a high-level baseball pitcher, tennis player, or golfer in slow motion? Most movements from the ground require the athlete to accelerate through a long compliant range of motion with high drive and quick deceleration capabilities of load to create a powerful whip-like motion through the torso. What sets these athletes apart is how mobile their bodies are, specifically the torso which would create low explode. If I ask a rotational athlete to run or jump effectively, it may appear as though they are not athletic or inefficient because many of the ground reaction forces are lost or dissipated through the compliant torso due to an inability to brace or create stiffness throughout the torso. This is the characteristic (high mobility in the spine) that facilitates rotatory power. When you run and jump effectively, it requires some level of posturing through the torso to stay erect. When you rely on torso compliance to swing or throw effectively, there is an inability to create stiffness. The mobility in the spine and compliance in the trunk musculature separates rotational athletes from lateral or linear athletes.

TRAINING MISCONCEPTIONS ABOUT THE ROTATIONAL ATHLETE

To ask a rotational athlete such as a golfer to react and jump like a basketball player is unrealistic. A rotational athlete cannot produce the amount of stiffness through the torso that is required of a sprinter, running back, or basketball player to run, jump or react effectively. A golfer needs compliance throughout the torso to swing with a great range of motion. On the other hand, to have a basketball player swing a golf club or tennis racquet, they may appear tight or immobile.

MAINTAINING THE ROTATIONAL ATHLETE IN-SEASON

Once a rotational athlete has been created with a combination of weight room exercises and the high volume of sport-specific reps (swinging and pitching) that occur during practice, the weight room focus should change to keep the athlete healthy and injury free. If the athlete becomes too mobile (hypermobile) through the torso, this could lead to injury. In this case, torso stiffness exercises would be needed. A program that prescribes anterior and posterior chain movements and involves posturing to protect the spine (dead lift, one-side loaded exercises) is recommended for the in-season prescription.

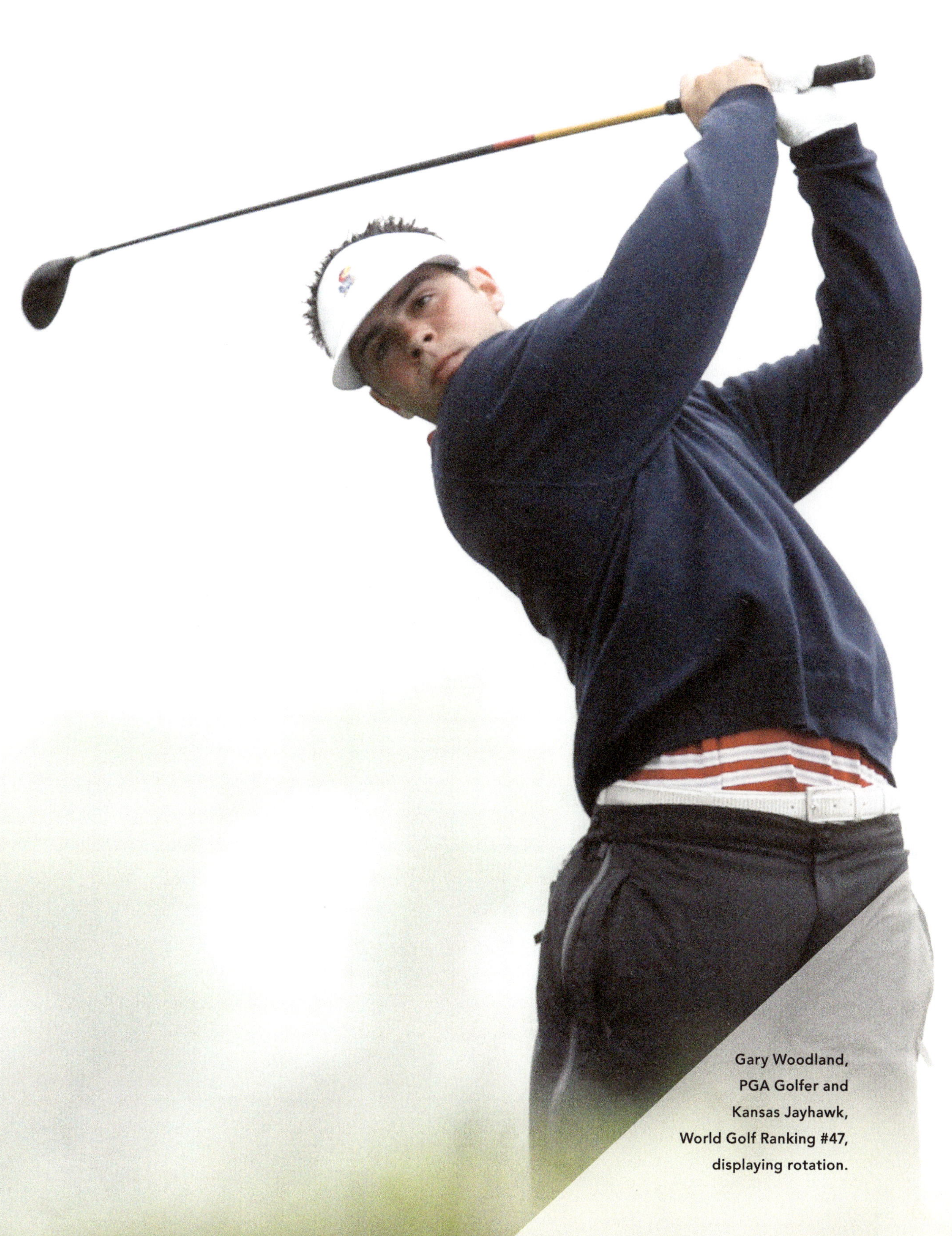

Gary Woodland,
PGA Golfer and
Kansas Jayhawk,
World Golf Ranking #47,
displaying rotation.

Year Round Training Concepts for the Rotational Athlete

When to Perform	Off Season	Pre Season	In Season	Post Season
Which Program	Rotational	Rotational	Lateral or Linear	Lateral or Linear
Purpose	Increase total power and anterior/posterior chain strength	Increase total power and anterior/posterior chain strength	Increase total power and anterior/posterior chain strength	Increase total power and anterior/posterior chain strength
	CREATE COMPLIANCE		MAINTAIN COMPLIANCE	
Movements	1° Long healthy movements to increase muscle compliance and joint mobility 2° High intensity rotational movements and complete range of motion	1° Long healthy movements to increase muscle compliance and joint mobility 2° High intensity rotational movements and complete range of motion	1° Short ballistic movements to increase joint stability and muscular stiffness to counteract long mobile powerful rotational movements 2° Bracing and posturing exercises	1° Short ballistic movements to increase joint stability and muscular stiffness to counteract long mobile powerful rotational movements 2° Bracing and posturing exercises
Emphasis	1° Strength (load- based resistance training) 2° Power (velocity-based resistance training)	1° Strength (load- based resistance training) 2° Power (velocity-based resistance training)	1° Power (velocity-based resistance training) 2° Strength (load- based resistance training)	1° Power (velocity-based resistance training) 2° Strength (load- based resistance training)

Movement Skills to Create the Rotational Athlete in the off-season & pre-season

(see movement skills in Section 5)

Position	Off season and pre season needs	Emphasis Long Response	Development	Movement	Action
Rotational	Posterior/ Anterior Chain Development	1° Speed Development 2° Long response plyometrics 3° Depth jump landing mechanics 4° Depth Jumps 5° Short response plyometrics 6° Agility	1° Compliance 2° Stiffness	1° Predetermined 2° Reactive	1° Accelerating 2° Braking

THE WORKOUTS: the Rotational Athlete

The following is a simple calendar that represents what a training month can look like.

ATHLETE
SAMPLE MONTHLY CALENDAR

SUNDAY	MONDAY	TUESDAY	WEDNESDAY	THURSDAY	FRIDAY	SATURDAY
	DAY 1	*MOVEMENT SKILLS*	**DAY 2**	*MOVEMENT SKILLS*	**DAY 3**	
	DAY 1	*MOVEMENT SKILLS*	**DAY 2**	*MOVEMENT SKILLS*	**DAY 3**	
	DAY 1	*MOVEMENT SKILLS*	**DAY 2**	*MOVEMENT SKILLS*	**DAY 3**	
	DAY 1	*MOVEMENT SKILLS*	**DAY 2**	*MOVEMENT SKILLS*	**DAY 3**	
	DAY 1	*MOVEMENT SKILLS*	**DAY 2**	*MOVEMENT SKILLS*	**DAY 3**	

The following pages contain workouts for the beginner, intermediate, advanced, and elite rotational athlete.

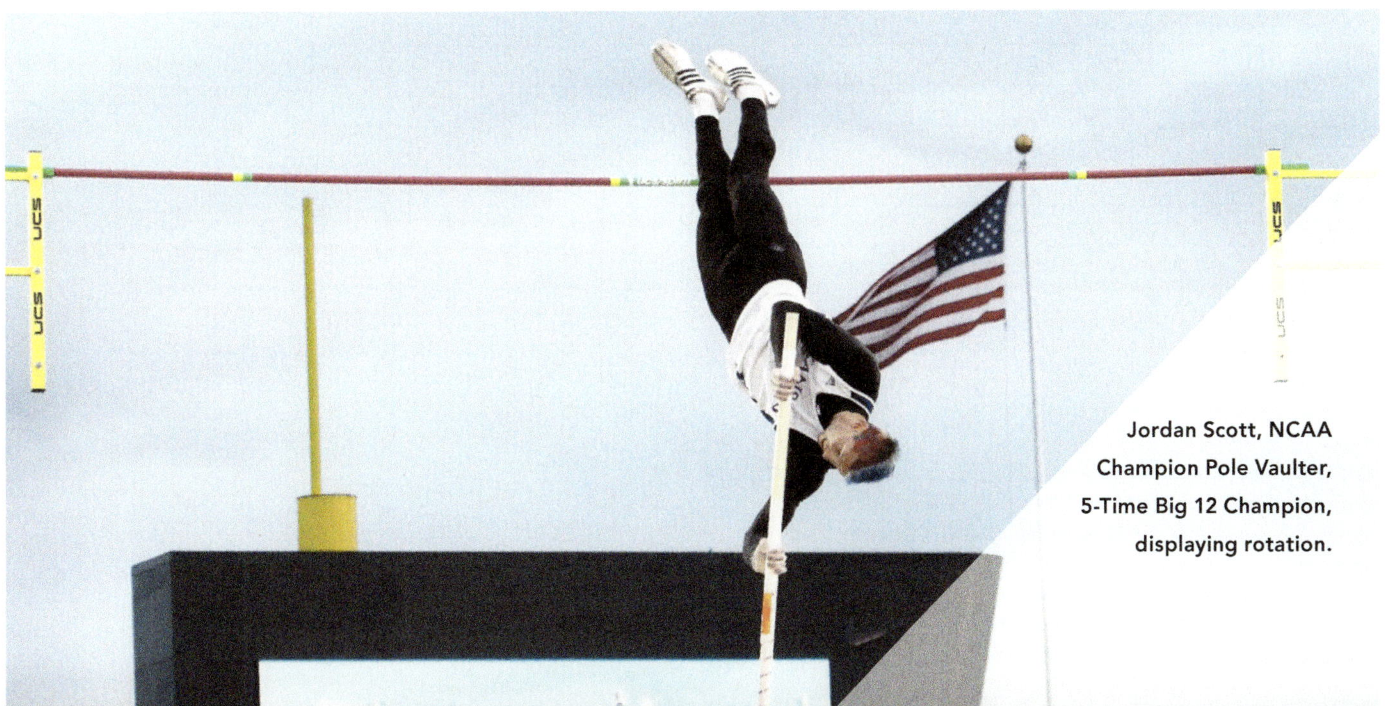

Jordan Scott, NCAA Champion Pole Vaulter, 5-Time Big 12 Champion, displaying rotation.

Eight Week Movement Plan for the Rotational Athlete (see movement skills in Section 5)								
	Week 1	**Week 2**	**Week 3**	**Week 4**	**Week 5**	**Week 6**	**Week 7**	**Week 8**
Speed Development (Sets)	**2 sets**	**2 sets**	**2 sets**	**2 sets**	**3 sets**	**3 sets**	**3 sets**	**3 sets**
Long Response Plyometrics								
6 inches								
Linear (Foot Contacts)	50	70	90	100				
Lateral (Foot Contacts)	12	16	20	25				
12 inches								
Linear (Foot Contacts)					50	70	90	100
Lateral (Foot Contacts)					12	16	20	25
Short Response Plyometrics								
6 inches								
Linear (Foot Contacts)	50	70	90	100				
Lateral (Foot Contacts)	12	16	20	25				
12 inches								
Linear (Foot Contacts)					50	70	90	100
Lateral (Foot Contacts)					12	16	20	25
Box Height (if applicable)	**12 inches**	**14 inches**	**16 inches**	**18 inches**	**22 inches**	**24 inches**	**28 inches**	**30 inches**
Box Jumps (Sets x Reps)	2 x 5	2 x 5	2 x 3	2 x 3	2 x 3	2 x 4	2 x 5	2 x 5
Landing Mechanics-Depth Jumps								
Sets x Reps	1 x 5	1 x 5	1 x 5	1 x 3				
Depth Jumps								
Sets x Reps					2x3	2 x 3	2 x 3	3x3
Predetermined Linear Patterns	10	12	15	16	20	22	25	28
(Total Reps)								
Agility Drills (Total Reps)	10	12	15	16	20	22	25	28

ROTATIONAL BEGINNER

Day 1 — Hypertrophy

Exercise	Sets	Reps	Purpose
A1) PVC OH Squat	3	6/6	Lower Body Anterior Chain/Mobility
A2) Cobra - Downward Dog - Child's Pose	3	10	Compliance
A3) Saigon Stretch	3	30 s	Compliance
B1) Back Extension	3	10	Lower Body Posterior Chain
B2) Pushup (Use Incline if Needed)	3	10/10	Upper Body Horizontal Push
B3) Warrior Stance	3	30 s	Compliance
C1) Walking Lunge	3	5/5	Lower Body Posterior Chain
C2) Figure 4 Stretch	3	30 s	Compliance
C3) Seated Row	3	8	Upper Body Horizontal Pull

Day 2 — Power

Exercise	Sets	Reps	Purpose
A1) Squat Jump	3	5	Total Body Explosive
A2) Lateral Windmill	3	8/8	Lateral Movement
A3) DB Incline Bench	3	5	Upper Body Vertical Push
B1) Burpee	3	4	Total Body Explosive/Stiffness/Mobility
B2) 1 Leg Glute Bridge	3	6/6	Lower Body Posterior Chain
B3) Lat Pulldown	3	6	Upper Body Vertical Pull
C1) Box Jump	3	4	Total Body Explosive
C2) Plate Torso Twist	3	6/6	Compliance
C3) PVC Over & Back	3	10/10	Compliance

Day 3 — Strength

Exercise	Sets	Reps	Purpose
A1) 1 Leg RDL	3	6/6	Lower Body Posterior Chain
A2) Alternating Spiderman	3	8/8	Compliance
A3) PVC Behind the Neck Press	3	8	Upper Body Horizontal Push/Compliance
B1) SB Leg Curl	3	8	Lower Body Posterior Chain
B2) PVC Seated Thoracic Twist	3	10/10	Compliance
B3) Pushup (Use Incline if Needed)	3	8	Upper Body Horizontal Push
C1) Squat	3	6	Lower Body Posterior Chain
C2) Inverted Row	3	8	Upper Body Horizontal Pull
C3) Cobra - Downward Dog - Child's Pose	3	5	Compliance

ROTATIONAL INTERMEDIATE

Day 1 — Hypertrophy

Exercise	Sets	Reps	Purpose
A1) Good Morning	4	10	Lower Body Posterior Chain
A2) Downward Dog - Cobra - Child's Pose	4	10	Compliance
A3) PVC Over & Back	4	10	Compliance
B1) Lateral Squat	4	8/8	Lower Body Posterior Chain/Mobility
B2) Alternating Spiderman	4	6/6	Compliance
B3) Lateral Raise	4	10	Upper Body Accessory
C1) Front Squat	4	8	Lower Body Anterior Chain
C2) Saigon Stretch	4	30 s	Compliance
C3) PVC Seated Thoracic Twist	4	10/10	Compliance

Day 2 — Power

Exercise	Sets	Reps	Purpose
A1) Split Squat	4	5/5	Lower Body Anterior Chain
A2) Pull Up	4	6	Upper Body Vertical Pull
A3) Warrior Stance	4	30 s	Compliance
B1) Glute Ham	4	4	Lower Body Posterior Chain
B2) Figure 4 Stretch	4	30 s	Compliance
B3) Foam Roll Calves	4	10/10	Compliance
C1) BB Hip Lift	4	5	Lower Body Posterior Chain
C2) Lateral Windmill	4	10/10	Lateral Movement
C3) DB OH Press	4	8	Upper Body Vertical Push

Day 3 — Strength

Exercise	Sets	Reps	Purpose
A1) Sumo Squat	4	6	Lower Body Posterior Chain
A2) MB OH Slam	4	5	Total Body Explosive
A3) DB Incline Bench Press	4	8	Upper Body Vertical Push
B1) Reverse X-Over Lunge	4	6/6	Lower Body Posterior Chain/Mobility
B2) DB Incline Row	4	8	Upper Body Vertical Pull
B3) Lateral Windmill	4	8/8	Lateral Movement
C1) Deadlift	4	6	Lower Body Posterior Chain
C2) 1 Leg Hip Lift	4	8/8	Lower Body Posterior Chain
C3) Alternating Spiderman	4	6/6	Compliance

ROTATIONAL ADVANCED

Day 1 Speed - Strength

Exercise	Sets	Reps	Purpose
A1) Jump Squat	3	5	Total Body Explosive
A2) PVC Seated Thoracic Twist	3	8/8	Compliance
A3) PVC Over & Back	3	8	Compliance
B1) Power Snatch	3	4	Total Body Explosive
B2) DB Lateral Squat	3	6/6	Lower Body Posterior Chain
B3) Foam Roll IT Bands	3	10/10	Compliance
C1) Hang Clean - Front Squat	4	3	Total Body Explosive
C2) Warrior Stance	3	30 s	Compliance
C3) 1 Arm DB OH Press	3	5/5	Upper Body Vertical Push/Stiffness

Day 2 Strength - Speed

Exercise	Sets	Reps	Purpose
A1) High Pull	3	4	Total Body Explosive
A2) Alternating Spiderman	3	6/6	Compliance
A3) Heel Elevated OH Squat	3	6	Lower Body Anterior Chain/Mobility
B1) Barbell Hip Lift	4	5	Lower Body Posterior Chain
B2) Foam Roll IT Bands	4	10/10	Compliance
B3) Cable Column Chest Fly	4	10	Upper Body Accessory
C1) Clean	4	2	Total Body Explosive
C2) 1 Arm DB Row	4	10/10	Upper Body Horizontal Pull
C3) Saigon Stretch	4	30 s	Compliance

Day 3 Strength

Exercise	Sets	Reps	Purpose
A1) Sumo Squat	3	6	Lower Body Posterior Chain
A2) PVC Seated Thoracic Twist	3	10/10	Compliance
A3) DB Incline Bench Press	3	8	Upper Body Vertical Push
B1) Reverse X-Over Lunge	3	6/6	Lower Body Posterior Chain/Mobility
B2) 1 Leg Hip Lift	3	10/10	Lower Body Posterior Chain
B3) Lateral Windmill	3	10/10	Lateral Movement
C1) Deadlift	3	8	Lower Body Posterior Chain
C2) PVC Behind the Neck Press	3	10	Upper Body Vertical Push/ Compliance
C3) DB Incline Row	3	10	Upper Body Vertical Pull

ROTATIONAL ELITE

Day 1 — Speed - Strength

Exercise	Sets	Reps	Purpose
A1) DB 1 Arm Snatch	4	4/4	Total Body Explosive/Stiffness
A2) Plyo Rotational Pull Up	4	3/3	Upper Body Vertical Pull/Stiffness/ Anterior Chain
A3) Heel Elevated OH Squat	4	5	Lower Body Anterior Chain/Mobility
B1) Hang High Pull	4	4	Total Body Explosive
B2) Behind the Neck Jerk	4	4	Upper Body Explosive Vertical Push/ Mobility
B3) PVC Seated Thoracic Twist	4	10/10	Compliance
C1) Hang Clean - Front Squat	4	3	Total Body Explosive/Anterior Chain
C2) Saigon Stretch	4	30 s	Compliance
C3) 1 Arm DB OH Press	4	5/5	Upper Body Vertical Push/Stiffness

Day 2 — Strength - Speed

Exercise	Sets	Reps	Purpose
A1) OH Bulgarian Split Squat	4	4/4	Lower Body Posterior Chain/Mobility
A2) Pushup	4	5	Upper Body Horizontal Push
A3) Cobra - Downward Dog - Child's Pose	4	5	Compliance
B1) DB Lateral Squat	4	5	Lower Body Posterior Chain/Mobility
B2) Power Clean	4	20 yds	Total Body Explosive
B3) Bent Over Row	4	10	Upper Body Horizontal Pull
C1) Snatch	4	2	Total Body Explosive
C2) Incline Bench Press	4	6	Upper Body Vertical Push
C3) Alternating Spiderman	4	10/10	Compliance

Day 3 — Strength

Exercise	Sets	Reps	Purpose
A1) Front Foot Elevated Bulgarian Split Squat	4	4/4	Lower Body Posterior Chain/Mobility
A2) Figure 4 Stretch	4	30 s	Compliance
A3) Bench Press	4	8	Upper Body Horizontal Push
B1) BB Split Squat	4	5/5	Lower Body Posterior Chain
B2) PVC Seated Thoracic Twist	4	8/8	Compliance
B3) Pull Up	4	8	Upper Body Vertical Pull
C1) Deadlift	4	6	Lower Body Posterior Chain
C2) PVC Over & Back	4	10	Compliance

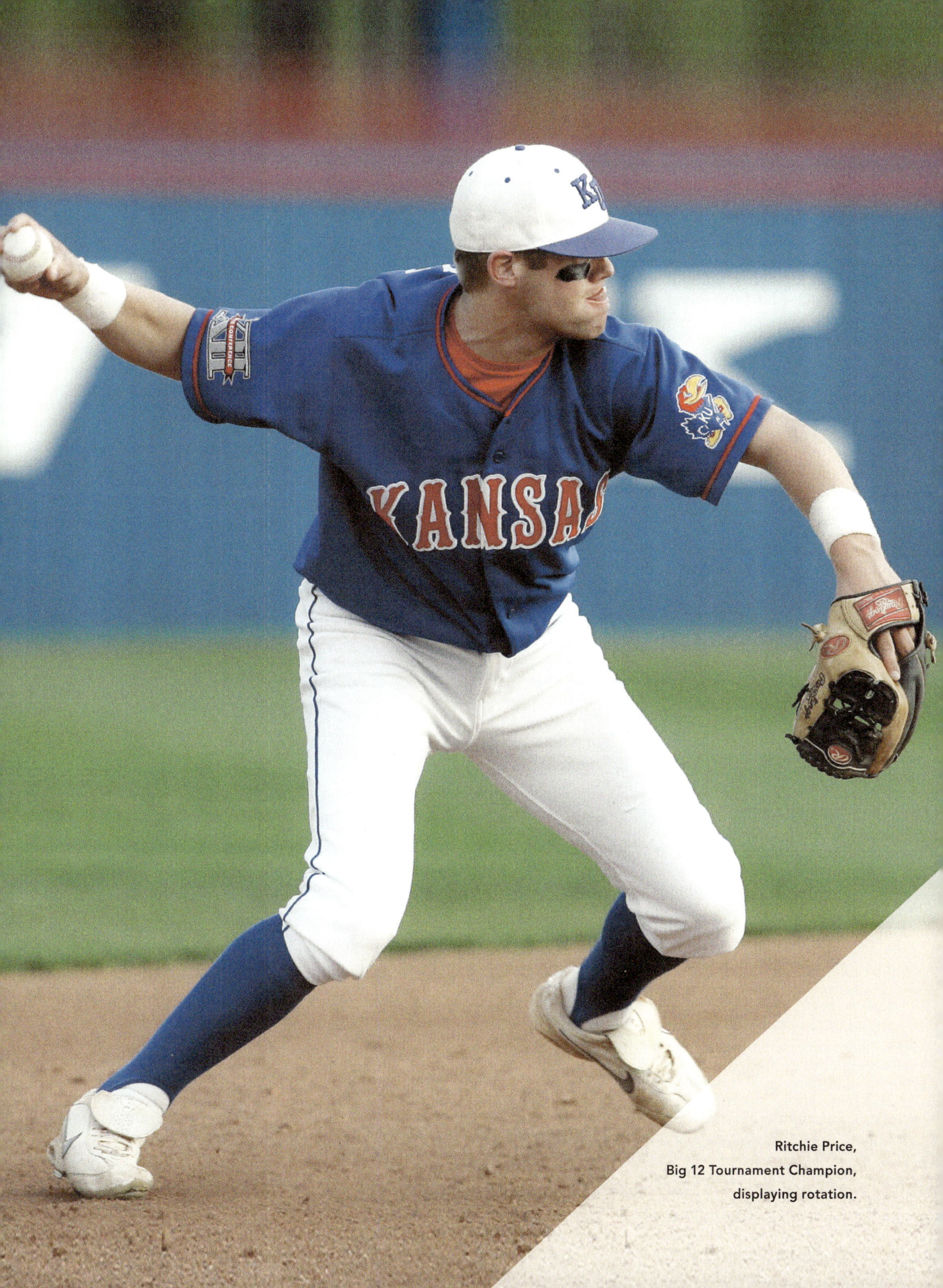

Ritchie Price,
Big 12 Tournament Champion,
displaying rotation.

SECTION 4: Defining the Linear Athlete

LINEAR ATHLETE FOR SPEED

Does the athlete run to reach top speed in a predetermined path in an event or sport? If you have ever watched a sprinter on the track, outside receiver, or safety on the football field, the athlete uses his entire foot while contacting the ground to reach top speed as opposed to the reactive athlete who primarily uses his forefoot to brake and change direction. This athlete has enough time to apply as much force into the ground through compliant posterior chain muscle contractions. The athlete knows where he is running or has a predetermined route that he is targeting. The healthy linear speed athlete uses a low amount of load or deceleration capabilities and has an ability to create stiffness (explode). What separates this athlete from the others is that he runs a predetermined path to top speed, therefore he has a high amount of drive.

Many of these ground reaction forces are being created through the athlete's posterior chain (ankle, knee and hips). In order to be efficient at sprinting, the athlete must also have torso stiffness to maintain a rigid, erect and efficient posture. Many coaches call this core strength.

TRAINING MISCONCEPTIONS ABOUT THE LINEAR ATHLETE FOR SPEED

To ask a sprinter or outside receiver to play basketball or defense would put him at a disadvantage because he is not trained to be reactive through anterior chain strength. If a sprinter is trained by doing agility drills and then is asked to sprint on the track, he will not be successful because he hasn't trained the posterior chain properly to sprint. Because the athlete hasn't been trained to reach top speed, there is also an increased risk of injury (hamstring strain) because the training wasn't specific. The athlete has been decelerating and performing agility drills instead of performing running a predetermined route and posterior chain exercises.

MAINTAINING THE LINEAR ATHLETE FOR SPEED IN-SEASON

Once the linear athlete has been created with a combination of weight room exercises and the high volume of sport-specific reps (sprinting drills and running patterns) that occur during practice, the weight room focus should change to keep the athlete healthy and injury free. The high intensity posterior chain muscle contractions must be offset with long and healthy anterior and posterior chain contractions while maintaining mobility in the weight room (rotational program). These specific prescriptions help the athlete stay mobile. To keep the athlete from overworking and fatiguing the posterior chain, prescribing a combination of compliant anterior chain (lateral), posterior chain, and mobility (lateral and rotational) exercises would be recommended for the in-season prescription.

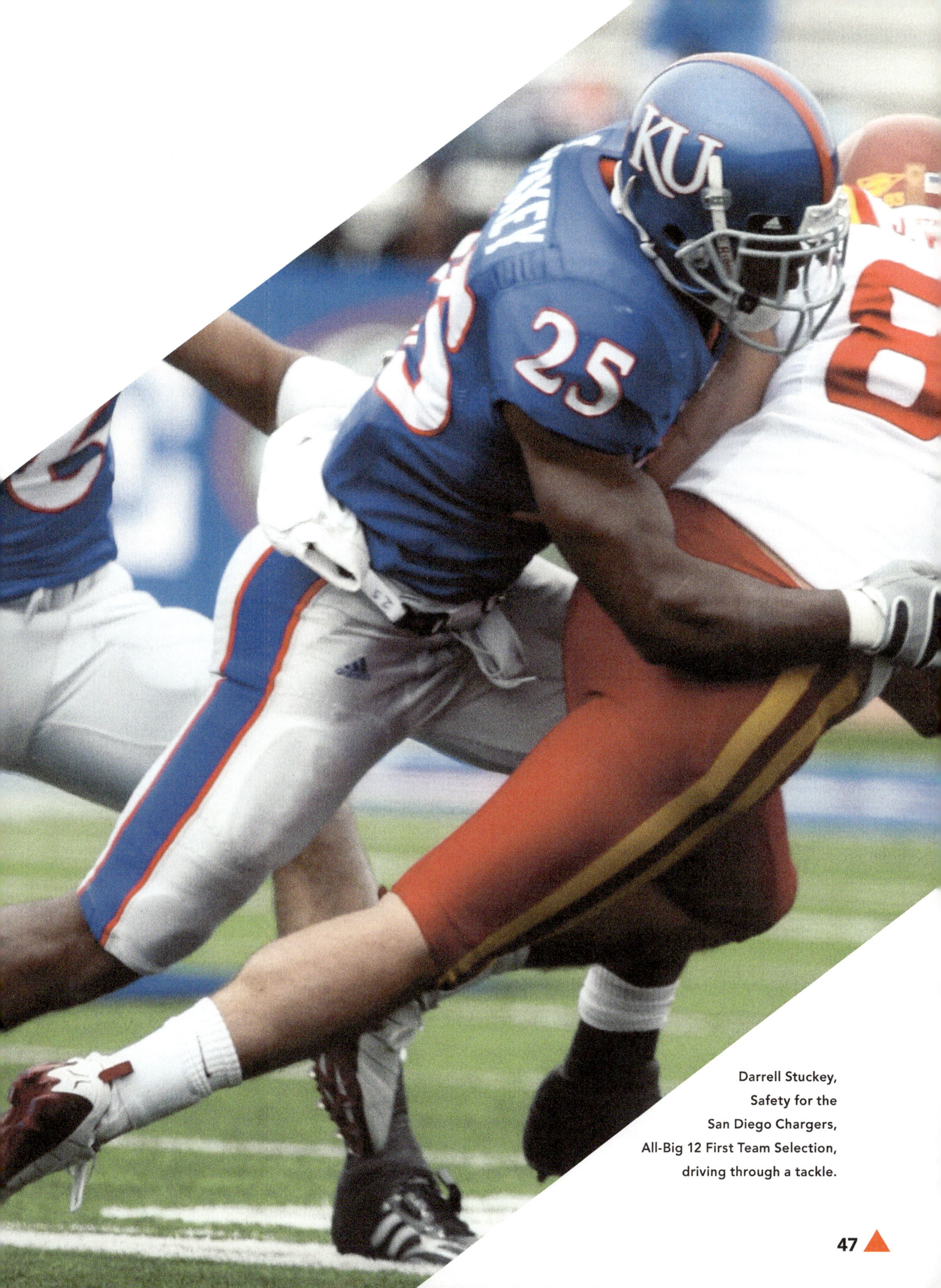

Darrell Stuckey,
Safety for the
San Diego Chargers,
All-Big 12 First Team Selection,
driving through a tackle.

Year Round Training Concepts for the Linear Speed Athlete

When to Perform	Off Season	Pre Season	In Season	Post Season
Which Program	Linear	Linear	Rotational or Lateral	Rotational or Lateral
Purpose	Increase total power and posterior chain strength	Increase total power and posterior chain strength	Increase total power and anterior chain strength	Increase total power and anterior chain strength
	CREATE COMPLIANCE & STIIFFNESS		MAINTAIN STIFFNESS & COMPLIANCE	
Movements	1° Long healthy movements to increase muscle compliance and joint mobility 2° Bracing and posturing exercises 3° Short ballistic movements to increase joint stability and muscular stiffness	1° Short ballistic movements to increase joint stability and muscular stiffness 2° Bracing and posturing exercises 3° Long healthy movements to increase muscle compliance and joint mobility	1° Counteract linear movements with lateral and rotational exercises 2° Long healthy movements to increase muscle compliance and joint mobility	1° Counteract linear movements with lateral and rotational exercises 2° Long healthy movements to increase muscle compliance and joint mobility
What	1° Strength (load- based resistance training) 2° Power (velocity-based resistance training)	1° Strength (load- based resistance training) 2° Power (velocity-based resistance training)	1° Power (velocity-based resistance training) 2° Strength (load- based resistance training)	1° Power (velocity-based resistance training) 2° Strength (load- based resistance training)

Movement Skills to Create the Linear Speed Athlete in the off-season & pre-season
(see movement skills in Section 5)

Position	Off season and pre season needs	Emphasis Long Response	Development	Movement	Action
Linear-Speed	1° Posterior Chain Development 2° Anterior Chain Development	1° Speed Development 2° Long response plyometrics 3° Box Jumps (up) 4° Short response plyometrics 5° Agility	1° Compliance 2° Stiffness	1° Predetermined 2° Reactive	1° Accelerating 2° Braking

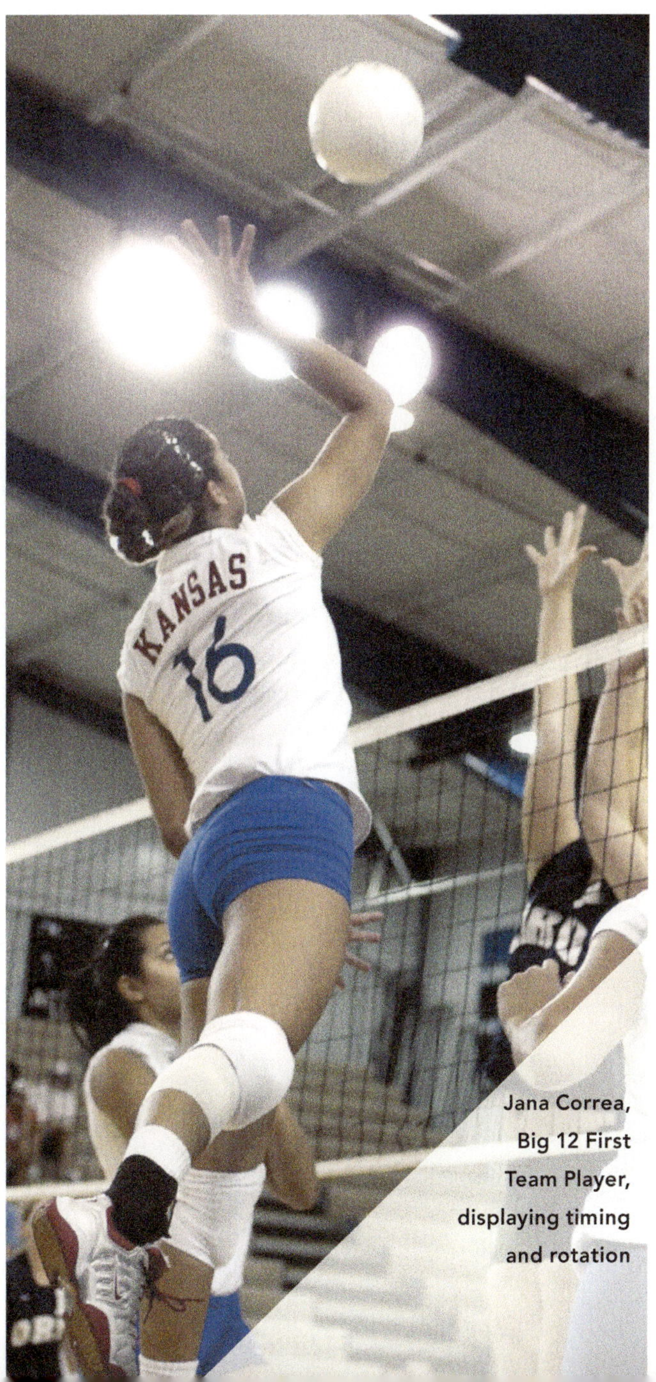

Jana Correa, Big 12 First Team Player, displaying timing and rotation

LINEAR ATHLETE FOR ENDURANCE

Have you ever watched a high level runner whose running is so efficient that it appears effortless? This athlete requires posturing abilities, torso stiffness, and posterior chain strength to be efficient. An endurance athlete does not want to waste energy with unwanted movements or instability in the torso. The endurance athlete's movements are rhythmical, repetitive, and methodical. The movement patterns are always the same. They are short and ballistic. The athlete becomes very stiff, yet very efficient, as a mover in their event or sport. To offset these patterns, lateral and mobility movements are important to stay compliant and healthy. The healthy linear athlete has a great ability to create stiffness, so explode is high. This athlete performs their sport in primarily a straight line; to excel at their sport requires them to have a low amount of load. In comparison with other athletes, this translates to a relatively low amount of strength but high performance.

TRAINING MISCONCEPTIONS ABOUT THE LINEAR ATHLETE FOR ENDURANCE

To ask an endurance athlete to be mobile is challenging because usually the stiffer an endurance athlete is, the more efficient they are. The activities that these athletes perform require many repetitions and hours of practice of doing the same thing. But there can come a time when too much stiffness can cause immobility or injury. In regards to exercise prescriptions, mobility exercises are what can keep the athlete healthy.

MAINTAINING THE LINEAR ATHLETE FOR ENDURANCE IN-SEASON

Once a stiff and efficient athlete has been created with a combination of weight room exercises and the high volume of sport-specific reps (running, swimming, and biking) that occur during practice, the weightroom focus should change to keep the athlete healthy and injury free. If the athlete becomes too stiff, mobility exercises would be needed because the athlete will be predisposed to muscle and joint injuries. A program that prescribes compliant anterior and posterior chain movements that involve mobility (offensive and rotational programs) is recommended for the in-season prescription.

Since the season is long for these types of athletes, there may be short periods of time when the athlete goes back to the pre season cycle to train through some competitions that are not as important as the competitions later in the season. Therefore, sometimes these athletes are not as concerned about where they place in competition and may 'train through' some competitions to increase performance for the end of the season competitions. This is where the training stimulus is more important than the competition stimulus.

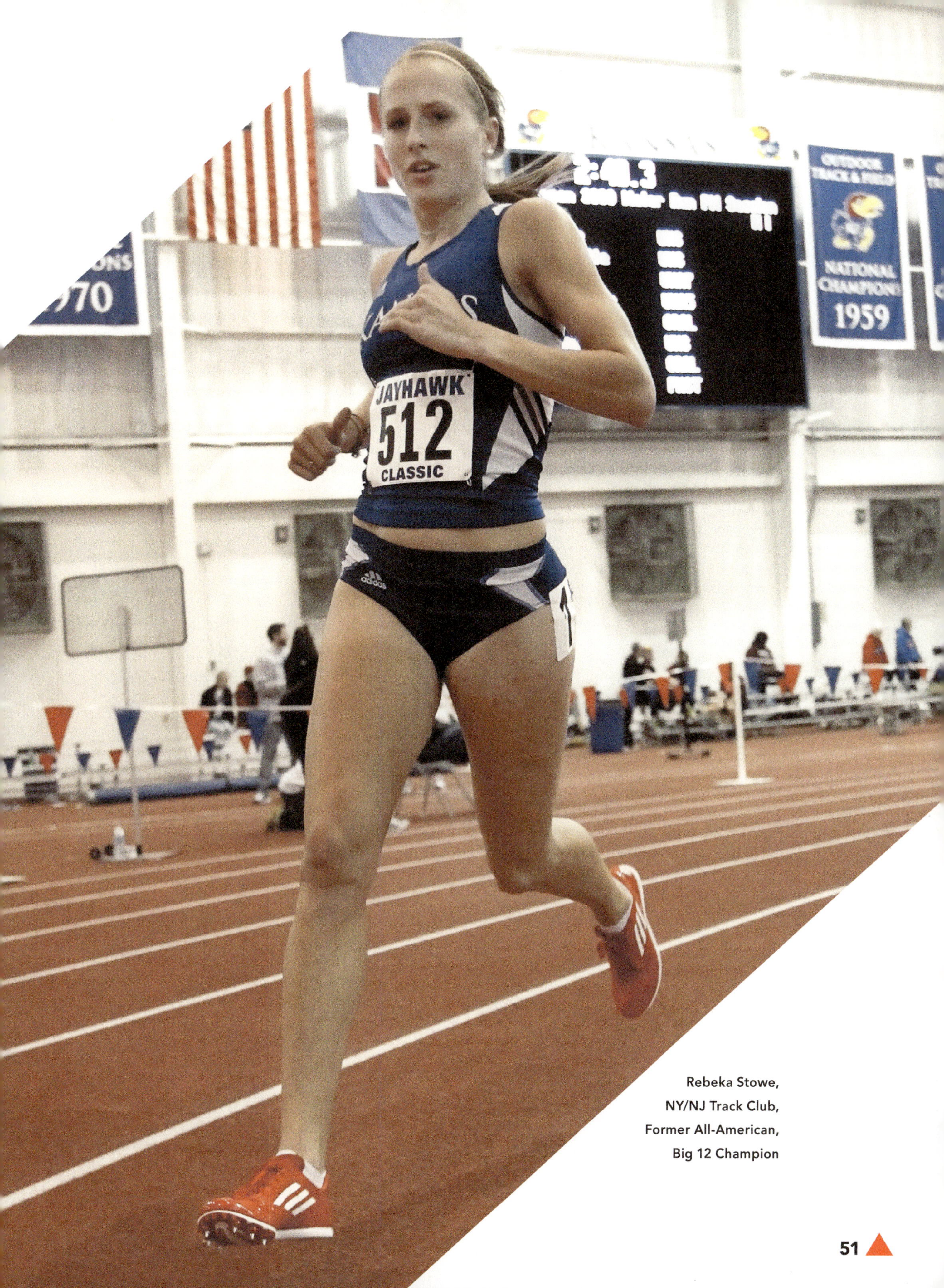

Rebeka Stowe,
NY/NJ Track Club,
Former All-American,
Big 12 Champion

Year Round Training Concepts for the Linear Endurance Athlete

When to Perform	Off Season	Pre Season	In Season	Post Season
Which Program	Rotational/Linear	Rotational/Linear	Rotational	Rotational
Purpose	Increase total power and anterior/posterior chain strength	Increase total power and anterior/posterior chain strength	Increase total power and anterior/posterior chain strength	Increase total power and anterior/posterior chain strength
	CREATE COMPLIANCE		MAINTAIN COMPLIANCE	
Movements	1° Long healthy movements to increase muscle compliance and joint mobility 2° Short ballistic movements to increase joint stability and muscular stiffness 3° Bracing and posturing exercises	1° Long healthy movements to increase muscle compliance and joint mobility 2° Short ballistic movements to increase joint stability and muscular stiffness 3° Bracing and posturing exercises	1° Long healthy movements to increase muscle compliance and joint mobility 2° Low intensity rotational movements and complete range of motion	1° Long healthy movements to increase muscle compliance and joint mobility 2° Low intensity rotational movements and complete range of motion
Emphasis	1° Strength (load- based resistance training) 2° Power (velocity-based resistance training)	1° Strength (load- based resistance training) 2° Power (velocity-based resistance training)	1° Power (velocity-based resistance training) 2° Strength (load- based resistance training)	1° Power (velocity-based resistance training) 2° Strength (load- based resistance training)

Movement Skills to Create the Linear Endurance Athlete in the off-season & pre-season

(see movement skills in Section 5)

Position	Off season and pre season needs	Emphasis Long Response	Development	Movement	Action
Linear-Endurance	Posterior/Anterior Chain Development	1° Speed Development 2° Long response plyometrics 3° Box Jumps (up) 4° Short response plyometrics 5° Agility	1° Stiffness 2° Compliance	1° Predetermined 2° Reactive	1° Accelerating 2° Braking

THE WORKOUTS: the Linear Athlete

The following is a simple calendar that represents what a training month can look like.

ATHLETE
SAMPLE MONTHLY CALENDAR

SUNDAY	MONDAY	TUESDAY	WEDNESDAY	THURSDAY	FRIDAY	SATURDAY
	DAY 1	*MOVEMENT SKILLS*	**DAY 2**	*MOVEMENT SKILLS*	**DAY 3**	
	DAY 1	*MOVEMENT SKILLS*	**DAY 2**	*MOVEMENT SKILLS*	**DAY 3**	
	DAY 1	*MOVEMENT SKILLS*	**DAY 2**	*MOVEMENT SKILLS*	**DAY 3**	
	DAY 1	*MOVEMENT SKILLS*	**DAY 2**	*MOVEMENT SKILLS*	**DAY 3**	
	DAY 1	*MOVEMENT SKILLS*	**DAY 2**	*MOVEMENT SKILLS*	**DAY 3**	

The following pages contain workouts for the beginner, intermediate, advanced, and elite linear athlete.

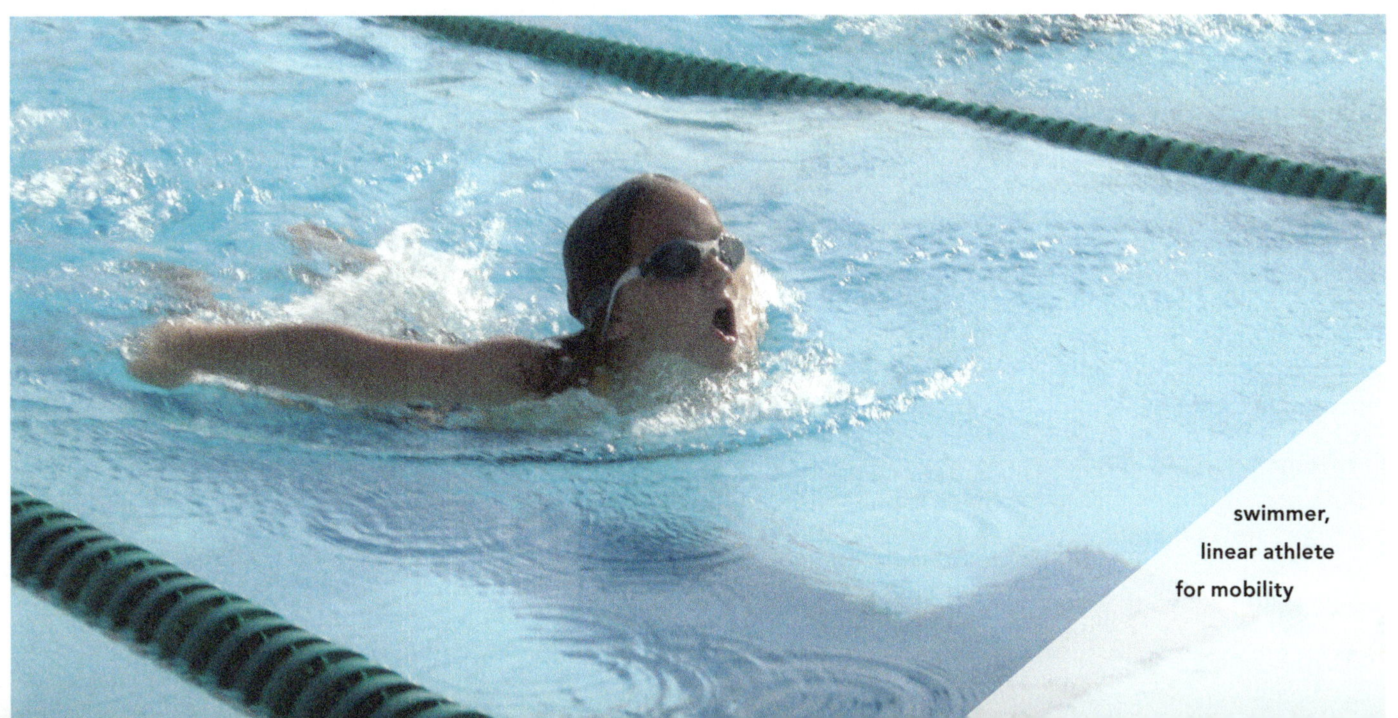

swimmer, linear athlete for mobility

Eight Week Movement Plan for the Linear Speed Athlete

(see movement skills in Section 5)

	Week 1	Week 2	Week 3	Week 4	Week 5	Week 6	Week 7	Week 8
Speed Development (Sets)	2 sets	2 sets	2 sets	2 sets	3 sets	3 sets	3 sets	3 sets
Long Response Plyometrics								
6 inches								
Linear (Foot Contacts)	100	140	180	200				
Lateral (Foot Contacts)	24	32	40	50				
12 inches								
Linear (Foot Contacts)					100	140	180	200
Lateral (Foot Contacts)					24	32	40	50
Box Height (if applicable)	12 inches	14 inches	16 inches	18 inches	22 inches	24 inches	28 inches	30 inches
Box Jumps (Sets x Reps)	3 x 5	3 x 5	4 x 3	4 x 3	4 x 3	4 x 2	4x2	4x2
Predetermined Linear Patterns (Total Reps)	20	25	30	35	40	45	50	55

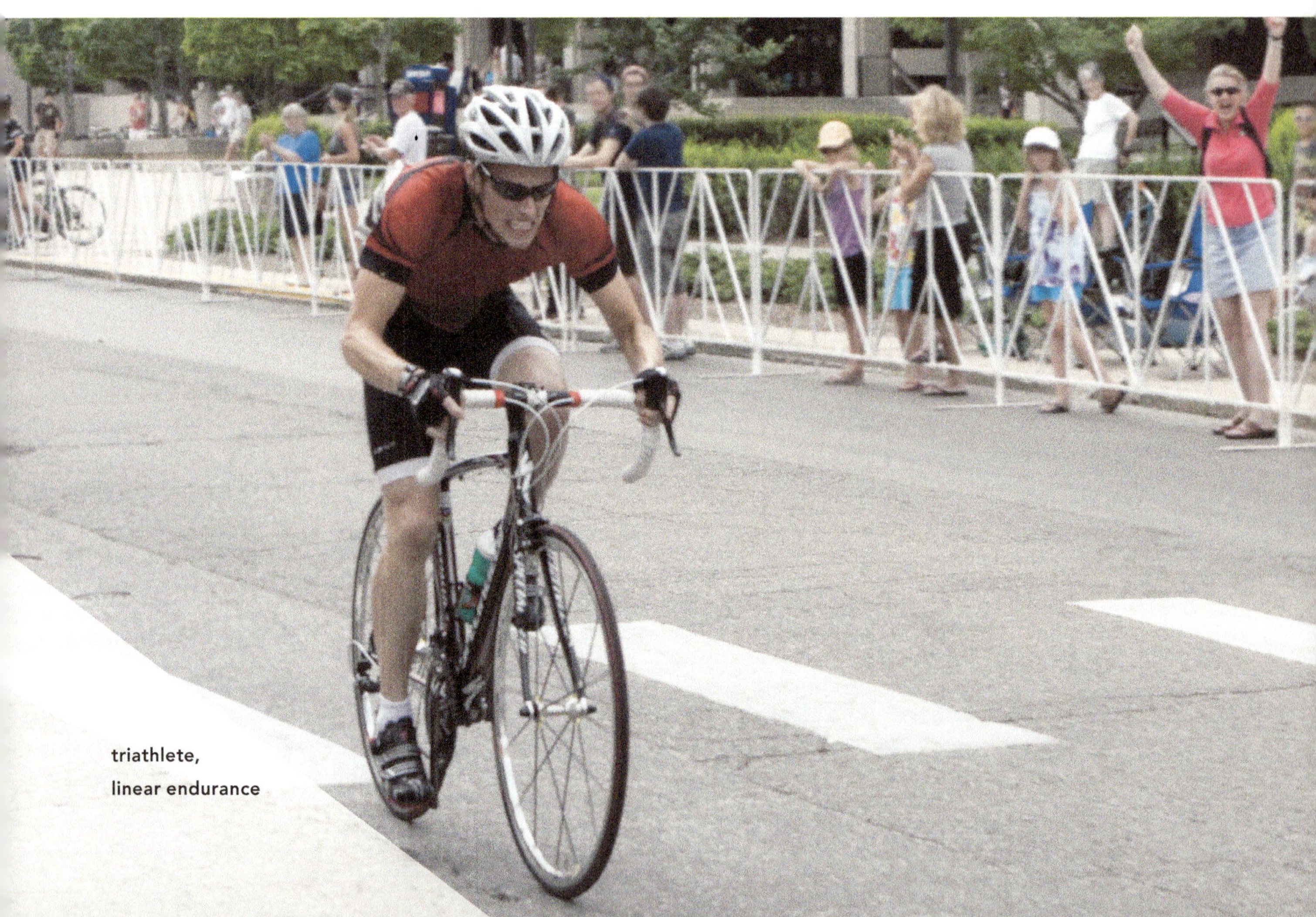

triathlete,
linear endurance

Eight Week Movement Plan for the Linear Endurance

(see movement skills in Section 5)

	Week 1	Week 2	Week 3	Week 4	Week 5	Week 6	Week 7	Week 8
Speed Development (Sets)	2 sets	2 sets	2 sets	2 sets	3 sets	3 sets	3 sets	3 sets
Long Response Plyometrics								
6 inches								
Linear (Foot Contacts)	25	35	45	50				
Lateral (Foot Contacts)	6	8	10	12				
12 inches								
Linear (Foot Contacts)					25	35	45	50
Lateral (Foot Contacts)					6	8	10	12
Short Response Plyometrics								
6 inches								
Linear (Foot Contacts)	25	35	45	50				
Lateral (Foot Contacts)	6	8	10	12				
12 inches								
Linear (Foot Contacts)					25	35	45	50
Lateral (Foot Contacts)					6	8	10	12
Box Height (if applicable)	12 inches	14 inches	16 inches	18 inches	22 inches	24 inches	28 inches	30 inches
Box Jumps (Sets x Reps)	2 x 5	2 x 5	2 x 3	2 x 3	2 x 3	2 x 4	2 x 5	2 x 5
Landing Mechanics-Depth Jumps								
Sets x Reps	1 x 5	1 x 5	1 x 5	1 x 3				
Depth Jumps								
Sets x Reps	1 x 5	1 x 5	1 x 3	2 x 2	3 x 3	2 x 3	2 x 3	2 x 3
Agility Drills (Reps)								
Acceleration	5	6	7	8	9	10	12	13
Deceleration	5	6	7	8	9	10	12	13

LINEAR BEGINNER

Day 1	Hypertrophy		
Exercise	**Sets**	**Reps**	**Purpose**
A1) Hip Lift	3	8	Lower Body Posterior Chain
A2) Figure 4 Stretch	3	30 s	Compliance
A3) Inverted Row	3	8	Upper Body Horizontal Pull
B1) Walking Lunge	3	6/6	Lower Body Posterior Chain
B2) Lateral Windmill	3	8/8	Lateral Movement
B3) Torso Twist	3	10/10	Compliance
C1) 1 Leg RDL	3	8/8	Lower Body Posterior Chain
C2) Lunge & Rotate	3	5/5	Lower Body Anterior Chain/Compliance
C3) Pushup (Use Incline if Needed)	3	10	Upper Body Horizontal Push

Day 2	Power		
Exercise	**Sets**	**Reps**	**Purpose**
A1) Squat Jump	3	5	Total Body Explosive
A2) Lateral Squat	3	5/5	Lower Body Posterior Chain/Mobility
A3) Saigon Stretch	3	20 s	Compliance
B1) Box Split Jump	3	3/3	Total Body Explosive/Anterior Chain
B2) Lat Pulldown	3	5	Upper Body Vertical Pull
B3) Alternating Spiderman	3	8/8	Compliance
C1) Burpee	3	4	Total Body Explosive/Stiffness/Mobility
C2) DB Incline	3	8	Upper Body Vertical Push

Day 3	Strength		
Exercise	**Sets**	**Reps**	**Purpose**
A1) Heel Elevated Squat	3	8	Lower Body Posterior Chain/Mobility
A2) Bench	3	8	Upper Body Horizontal Push
A3) Foam Roll Calves	3	10/10	Compliance
B1) Reverse X-Over Lunge	3	5/5	Lower Body Posterior Chain/Mobility
B2) Seated Row	3	8	Upper Body Horizontal Pull
C1) Glute Ham	3	6	Lower Body Posterior Chain
C2) DB OH Press	3	8	Upper Body Vertical Push
C3) Cobra - Downward Dog - Child's Pose	3	6	Compliance

LINEAR INTERMEDIATE

Day 1	Hypertrophy		
Exercise	**Sets**	**Reps**	**Purpose**
A1) DB 1 Leg RDL	4	8/8	Lower Body Posterior Chain
A2) DB OH Press	4	10	Upper Body Vertical Push
A3) Alternating Spiderman	4	10/10	Compliance
B1) BB Bulgarian Split Squat	4	6/6	Lower Body Posterior Chain/Mobility
B2) 1 Arm DB Row	4	10/10	Upper Body Horizontal Pull
B3) PVC Seated Thoracic Twist	4	8/8	Compliance
C1) Back Squat	4	8	Lower Body Posterior Chain
C2) Foam Roll Calves	4	10/10	Compliance

Day 2	Strength		
Exercise	**Sets**	**Reps**	**Purpose**
A1) 1 Leg Glute Bridge	4	6/6	Lower Body Posterior Chain
A2) Foam Roll IT Bands	4	10/10	Compliance
B1) BB Hip Lift	4	6	Lower Body Posterior Chain
B2) Leg Swings Forward/Backwards	4	8/8	Compliance
B3) Bench Press	4	6	Upper Body Horizontal Push
C1) Deadlift	4	8	Lower Body Posterior Chain
C2) Leg Swings Left/Right	4	8/8	Compliance
C3) Seated Row	4	6	Upper Body Horizontal Pull

Day 3	Muscle Power		
Exercise	**Sets**	**Reps**	**Purpose**
A1) Heel Elevated OH Squat	4	5	Lower Body Anterior Chain/Mobility
A2) Lateral Squat	4	5/5	Lower Body Posterior Chain/Mobility
A3) Saigon Stretch	4	40 s	Compliance
B1) Box Jump	4	5	Total Body Explosive
B2) DB Incline Bench Press	4	8	Upper Body Vertical Push
C1) Split Squat	4	4/4	Lower Body Posterior Chain/Mobility
C2) Lat Pulldown	4	8	Upper Body Vertical Pull
C3) Figure 4 Stretch	4	40 s	Compliance

LINEAR ADVANCED

Day 1	Speed - Strength		
Exercise	**Sets**	**Reps**	**Purpose**
A1) Good Morning	4	5	Lower Body Posterior Chain
A2) Incline Bench Press	4	8	Upper Body Vertical Push
A3) Foam Roll Calves	4	10/10	Compliance
B1) Power Snatch	4	4	Total Body Explosive
B2) Lat Pulldown	4	8	Upper Body Vertical Pull
B3) PVC Seated Thoracic Twist	4	8/8	Compliance
C1) Hang Clean - Front Squat	4	5	Total Body Explosive/Anterior Chain
C2) Foam Roll IT Bands	4	10/10	Compliance

Day 2	Strength - Speed		
Exercise	**Sets**	**Reps**	**Purpose**
A1) Clean Pull	4	4	Total Body Explosive
A1) Bulgarian Split Squat	4	10/10	Compliance
B1) OH Drop Squat	4	3	Lower Body Anterior Chain/Mobility
B2) Clean	4	2	Total Body Explosive
B3) DB Bench Press	4	8	Upper Body Horizontal Push
C1) BB Hip Lift	4	5	Lower Body Posterior Chain
C2) Alternating Spiderman	4	8/8	Compliance
C3) Seated Row	4	6	Upper Body Horizontal Pull

Day 3	Strength		
Exercise	**Sets**	**Reps**	**Purpose**
A1) Heel Elevated OH Squat	4	6	Lower Body Anterior Chain/Mobility
A2) Swiss Ball Leg Curl	4	6	Lower Body Posterior Chain
A3) Foam Roll Hamstrings/Glutes	4	30 s	Compliance
B1) RDL	4	5	Lower Body Posterior Chain
B2) Incline Bench Press	4	8	Upper Body Vertical Push
C1) Deadlift	4	6	Lower Body Posterior Chain
C2) Pull Up	4	8	Upper Body Vertical Pull
C3) Foam Roll Quads	4	10/10	Compliance

LINEAR ELITE

Day 1	Speed - Strength		
Exercise	**Sets**	**Reps**	**Purpose**
A1) Swiss Ball 1 Leg Curl	4	5/5	Lower Body Posterior Chain
A2) Seated Row	4	8	Upper Body Horizontal Pull
A3) Lateral Windmill	4	10/10	Compliance
B1) Power Jerk	4	3	Upper Body Vertical Push
B2) Box Jump	4	4	Total Body Explosive
B3) Alternating Spiderman	4	8/8	Compliance
C1) Hang Clean - Front Squat	4	5	Total Body Explosive/Anterior Chain
C2) Pull Up	4	5	Upper Body Vertical Pull

Day 2	Strength - Speed		
Exercise	**Sets**	**Reps**	**Purpose**
A1) OH Drop Squat	4	3	Lower Body Anterior Chain/Mobility
A2) OH Bulgarian Split Squat	4	5/5	Lower Body Posterior Chain/Mobility
B1) Hang Snatch	4	4	Total Body Explosive
B2) Bench Press	4	6	Upper Body Horizontal Push
B3) Lateral Squat	4	4/4	Lower Body Posterior Chain
C1) Clean Pull	4	2	Total Body Explosive
C2) Warrior Stance	4	30s	Compliance
C3) Lat Pulldown	4	6	Upper Body Vertical Pull

Day 3	Strength		
Exercise	**Sets**	**Reps**	**Purpose**
A1) BB 1 Leg Squat	4	6/6	Lower Body Anterior Chain/Stiffness
A2) BB Hip Lift	4	6/6	Lower Body Posterior Chain
A3) Saigon Stretch	4	30 s	Compliance
B1) OH Squat	4	5	Lower Body Posterior Chain/Mobility
B2) DB Incline Bench Press	4	8	Upper Body Vertical Push
C1) Deadlift	4	6	Lower Body Posterior Chain
C2) Seated Row	4	8	Upper Body Horizontal Pull
C3) Figure 4 Stretch	4	30 s	Compliance

SECTION 5: Movement Skills

This section will help you identify and incorporate the movement skills that are appropriate for each power position. These skills include speed development, continuous short response and continuous long response plyometrics, depth jumps, and agility drills to create the explosive athlete. These movement skills are specific to an athlete's movement needs as they prepare for the competitive season. Movement drills can be performed prior to the resistance training session or by themselves two to three times per week.

The following are terms that should be understood:

- **Speed Development** – To advance the ability to perform successive movements at a fast rate.
- **Run** – Alternating right and left leg ground contact.
- **Skip** – Same leg touches the ground consecutively then the other leg repeats pattern.
- **Hop** – Unilateral (1 leg) movement that causes displacement.
- **Jump** – Bilateral (2 leg) movement that causes displacement.
- **Plyometrics** – any continuous hop or jump.
- **Short response plyometrics** – Short ground time between continuous jumps/hops. These movements are quick and reactive through the forefoot. Relatively small changes in joint range of motions as the athlete accelerates and decelerates. These movements emphasize quickness.
- **Long response plyometrics** – Long ground time between continuous jumps/hops. These movements are slightly longer and more deliberate with the whole foot contacting the ground. Relatively large changes in joint range of motions as the athlete accelerates and decelerates. These movements are more deliberate and have slightly longer ground contact time.
- **Depth Jumps** – Jumping/hopping off a box then maximally jumping/hopping vertically after landing.
- **Agility** – The ability to change direction.

The hardest thing that a sports performance coach can do is prescribe workouts for athletes that they do not coach every day. The following skills are based on technique and progressions. If the athlete is not ready to progress based on walking, skipping, running, hopping, and jumping technique; keep them at their current level until technique, strength, and/or power are developed. The emphasis should be on the proper mechanics of acceleration/triple extension and landing mechanics/triple flexion:

1. Toes point forward
2. Knees track over toes
3. Torso stays upright

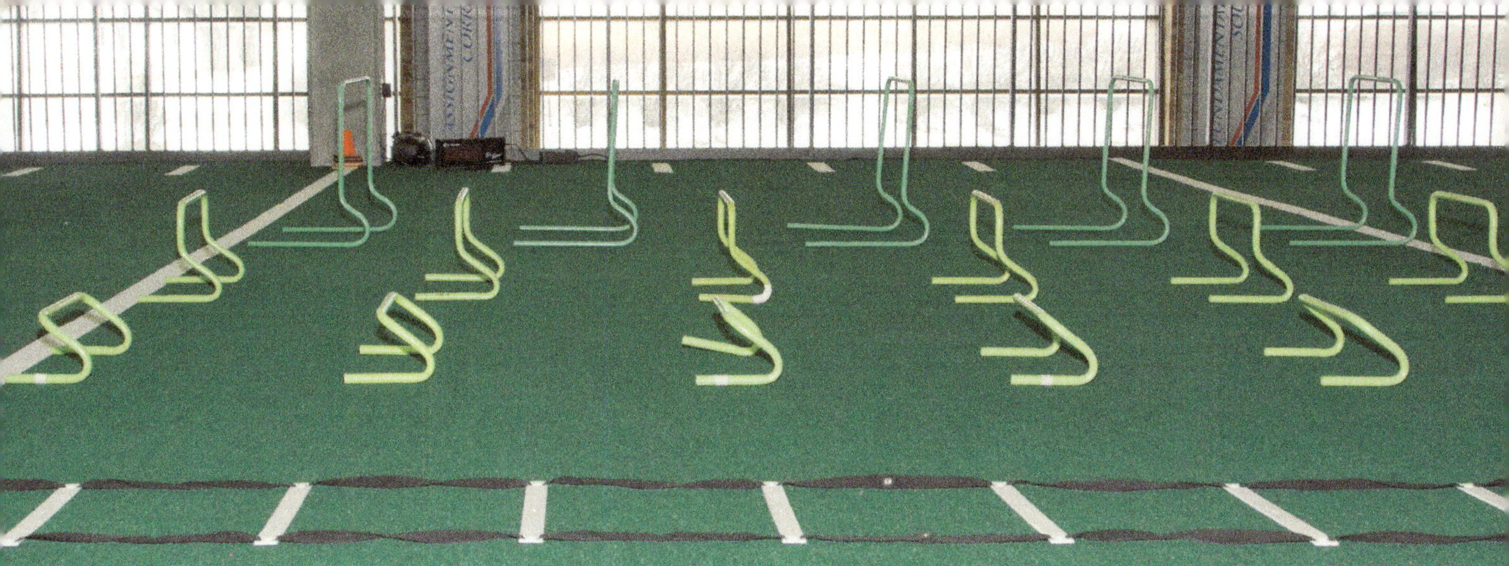

SPEED DEVELOPMENT SET

AGILITY LADDER (complete 10 reps of each exercise)

WALK

- Walking knee hug
- Walking toy soldier
- Walking quad walk
- Walking figure 4
- Walking lateral lunge

SKIP

- High knee skip
- Toy soldier skip
- Heel to hamstring skip
- Right and left dead leg single leg skip

RUN

- High knee run
- Straight leg stride
- Hamstring kick run

6 INCH MINI HURDLES (10 hurdles)

RUN

- Linear run over hurdles
- Right and left side lateral run over hurdles

12 INCH MINI HURDLES (10 hurdles)

RUN

- Linear run over hurdles
- Right and left side lateral run over hurdles

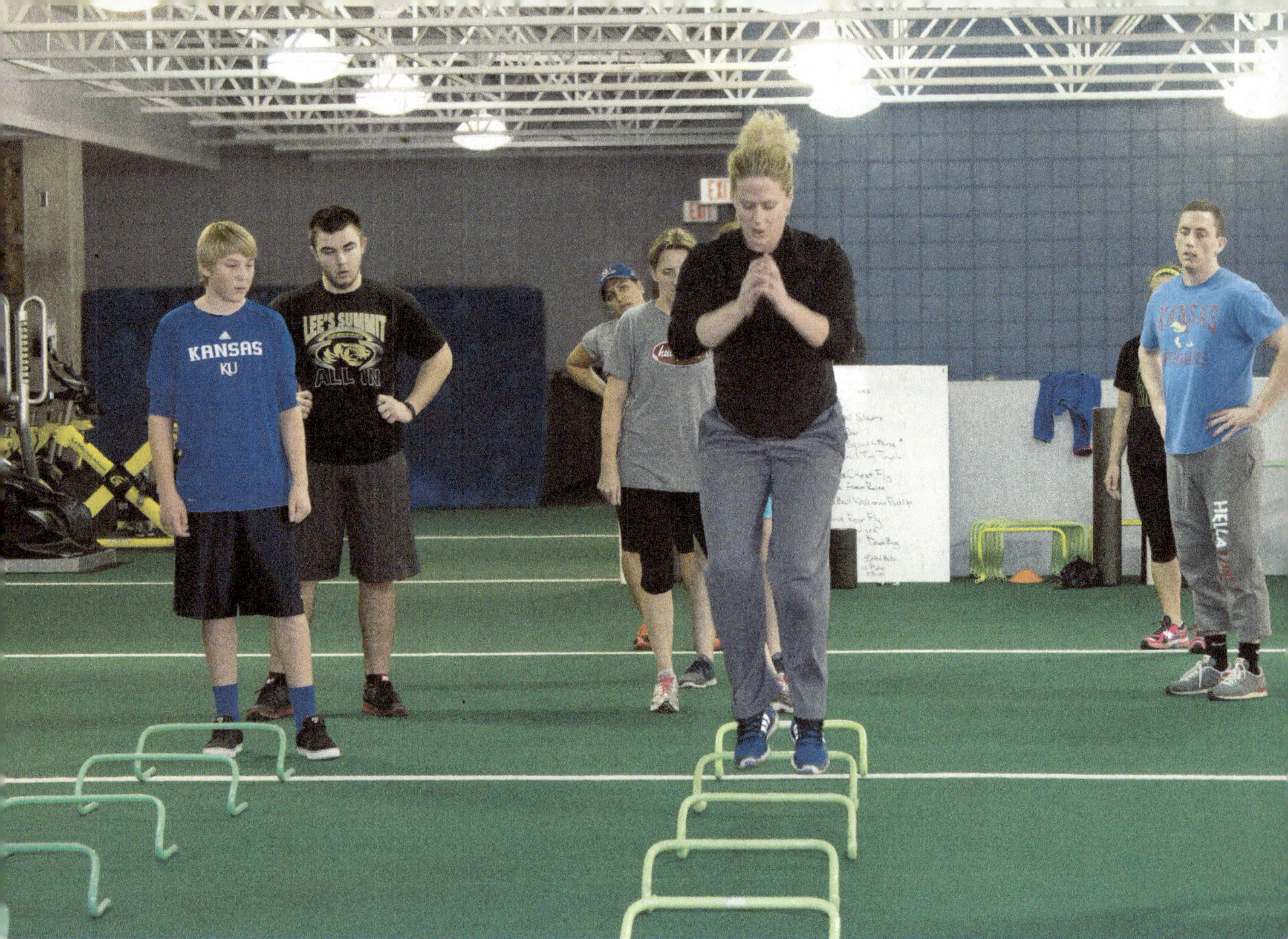

PLYOMETRICS

When performing short and long response plyometrics, the exercises look similar, but the **movement emphasis** determines the purpose. The purpose of short response plyometrics would be to develop more efficient anterior chain stiffness and reactivity. The purpose of the long response plyometrics would be to develop more compliant acceleration through the posterior chain.

SHORT RESPONSE PLYOMETRICS

Short ground response time between continuous jumps/hops. Relatively small changes in joint range of motions as the athlete accelerates and decelerates. It is quick with its movements. There are small joint angle changes. The athlete will primarily be anterior loaded on the forefoot.

LONG RESPONSE PLYOMETRICS

Long ground response time between continuous jumps/hops. Relatively large changes in joint range of motions as the athlete accelerates and decelerates. The greater changes in joint range of motions cause longer ground contact time as this ensures the whole foot touches the ground.

LINEAR

AGILITY LADDER

- Right and left single leg hops
- 2 leg jumps

6 INCH MINI HURDLES

2 leg rhythm jumps in series (jump over hurdle, low intensity recovery jump (rhythm jump to reset body position) to decrease transitional force, then jump over next hurdle, low intensity recovery jump (rhythm jump) to decrease transitional force x repeat 10 times)

- 1 hurdle
- 2 hurdles (if you have 10 hurdles this would be 5 jumps with a rhythm jump in between hurdles)
- 3 hurdles (if you have 10 hurdles this would be 3 jumps with a rhythm jump in between hurdles)

Jump (with no rhythm jump) over hurdles in series

- 1 hurdle
- 2 hurdles (if you have 10 hurdles this would be 5 jumps)
- 3 hurdles (if you have 10 hurdles this would be 3 jumps)

Right and left single leg hops in series

- 1 hurdle
- 2 hurdles

12 INCH MINI HURDLES

2 leg rhythm jumps in series (jump over hurdle, low intensity recovery jump (rhythm jump to reset body position) to decrease transitional force, then jump over next hurdle, low intensity recovery jump (rhythm jump) to decrease transitional force x repeat 10 times)

- 1 hurdle
- 2 hurdles (if you have 10 hurdles this would be 5 jumps with a rhythm jump in between hurdles)
- 3 hurdles (if you have 10 hurdles this would be 3 jumps with a rhythm jump in between hurdles)

Jump (with no rhythm jump) over hurdles in series

- 1 hurdle
- 2 hurdles (if you have 10 hurdles this would be 5 jumps)
- 3 hurdles (if you have 10 hurdles this would be 3 jumps)

Right and left single leg hops in series

- 1 hurdle
- 2 hurdles

LATERAL

6 INCH MINI HURDLES

(Only use 3 hurdles for these drills.
Jump over the hurdles and return over the same hurdles)

Right and left 2 leg jumps in series

- 1 hurdle (3 hurdles set up. Up and back is 6 jumps)

Right and left 1 leg hurdle

- 1 hurdle (3 hurdles set up. Up and back is 6 jumps)

12 INCH MINI HURDLES

Right and left 2 leg jumps in series

- 1 hurdle (3 hurdles set up. Up and back is 6 jumps)

Right and left 1 leg hurdle

- 1 hurdle (3 hurdles set up. Up and back is 6 jumps)

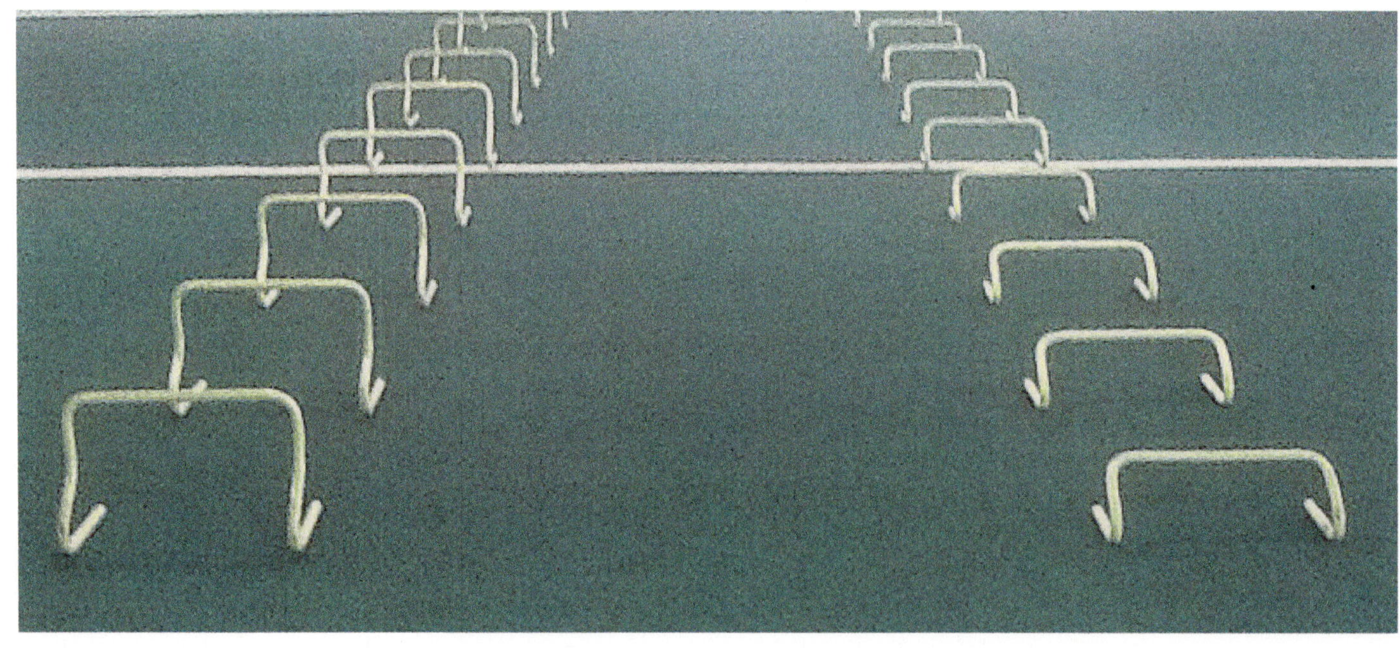

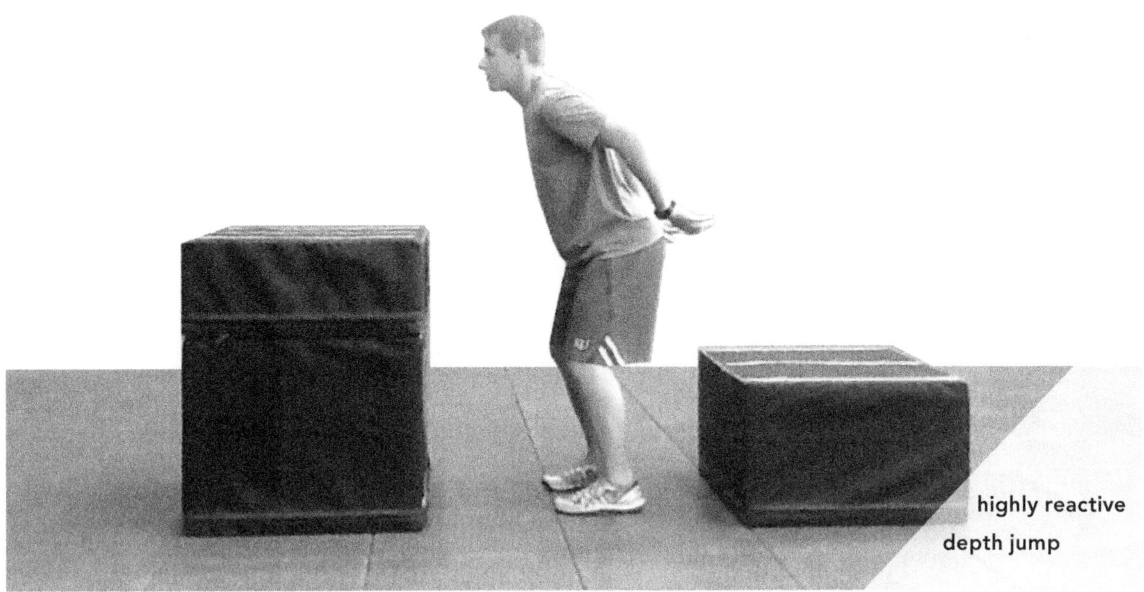

DEPTH JUMP DRILLS

1. Hopping/jumping **off** a box for landing mechanics
2. Hopping/jumping **off** a box then maximal vertical jump

   **Landing should be balanced and have 1 full solid contact as there should be no shifting or shuffling of the feet. Shifting the foot left to right and back and forth after landing shows that the athlete cannot handle the forces for proper deceleration. To correct this, use coaching cues or get a shorter box. A general range for plyometric boxes can be from 12 inches to 30 inches tall.

LINEAR

- 2 leg depth jump-stick landing to practice deceleration techniques
- 2 leg depth jump-after landing maximal jump for height
- Rapid fire 2 leg depth jumps on and off the box
- Right and left 1 leg depth jump-stick landing to practice deceleration techniques
- Right and left leg depth jump-after landing maximal jump for height

LATERAL

- Rapid fire right and left lateral double leg off and on box
- Rapid fire right and left lateral single leg off and on box

AGILITY DRILLS

LATERAL

ACCELERATION

- Lateral shuffle 10 yards
- Shuffle 5 yards, sprint 5 yards
- Shuffle 5 yards, backpedal 5 yards
- Carioca 10 yards

DECELERATION

- Right shuffle 5 yards, left shuffle back 5 yard
- Right carioca 5 yards, left carioca back 5 yard
- Right crossover step 5 yard, left crossover step back 5 yards

LINEAR

ACCELERATION

- Accelerate 10 yards
- Accelerate 5 yards, backpedal 5 yards
- Backpedal 10 yards
- Backpedal 5 yards, sprint 5 yards
- Carioca 10 yards

DECELERATION

- Accelerate 5 yards, touch line, back pedal 5 yards back
- Accelerate 5 yards, turn, and accelerate 5 yards back
- Backpedal 5 yards, touch line, sprint 5 yards

***Add any variation to progress to specific sport or position starts, i.e., changes in vertical agility (ex. push-up or back to ground start, end drill with vertical jump, or slide), rotational agility, lateral agility, or linear agility

Other variations can be as follows:

- React to implement (ball or noise)
- Add rotations
- 180 degree
- 360 degree

SECTION 6: Conclusion

The ability to produce force is the foundation on which athletes are built. The sequencing of force production from the feet and through the body makes an athlete different and able to excel at his position. It is the reason why a reactive basketball player is not as good at a fluid rotatory skill that a tennis or golf athlete has. It is why a pitcher or ice hockey player is not a quick and reactive jumper or sprinter like a defensive back. An athlete who is too loose or compliant in the torso when they sprint would need stiffening exercises to increase efficiency. A long distance runner who is too stiff and injury prone would need exercises to become more mobile and compliant to stay healthy.

To build the desired athlete, the exercise prescription should focus on the specific force production and sequencing required for the position. Once that position is created, the goal should be to maintain and build a healthier position-specific athlete.

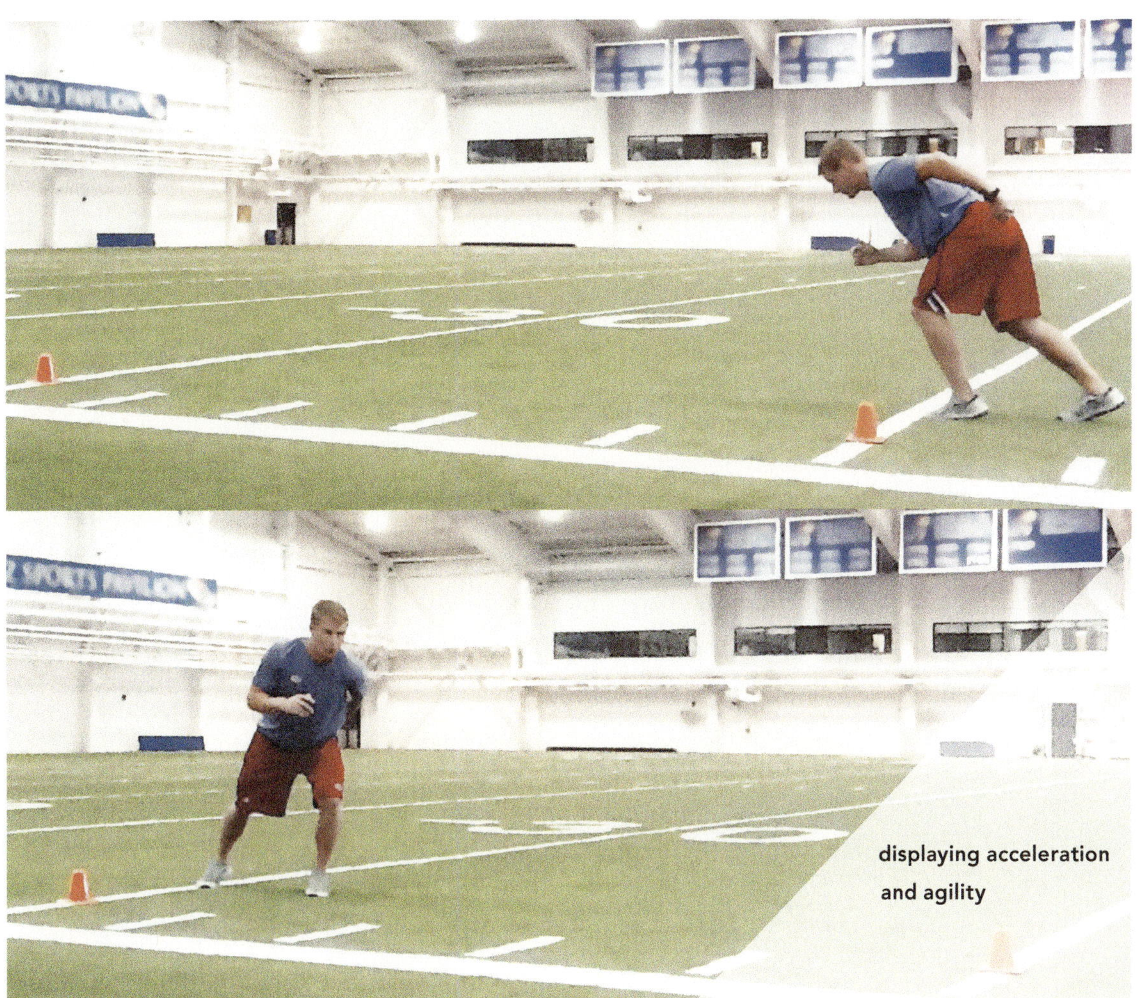

displaying acceleration and agility

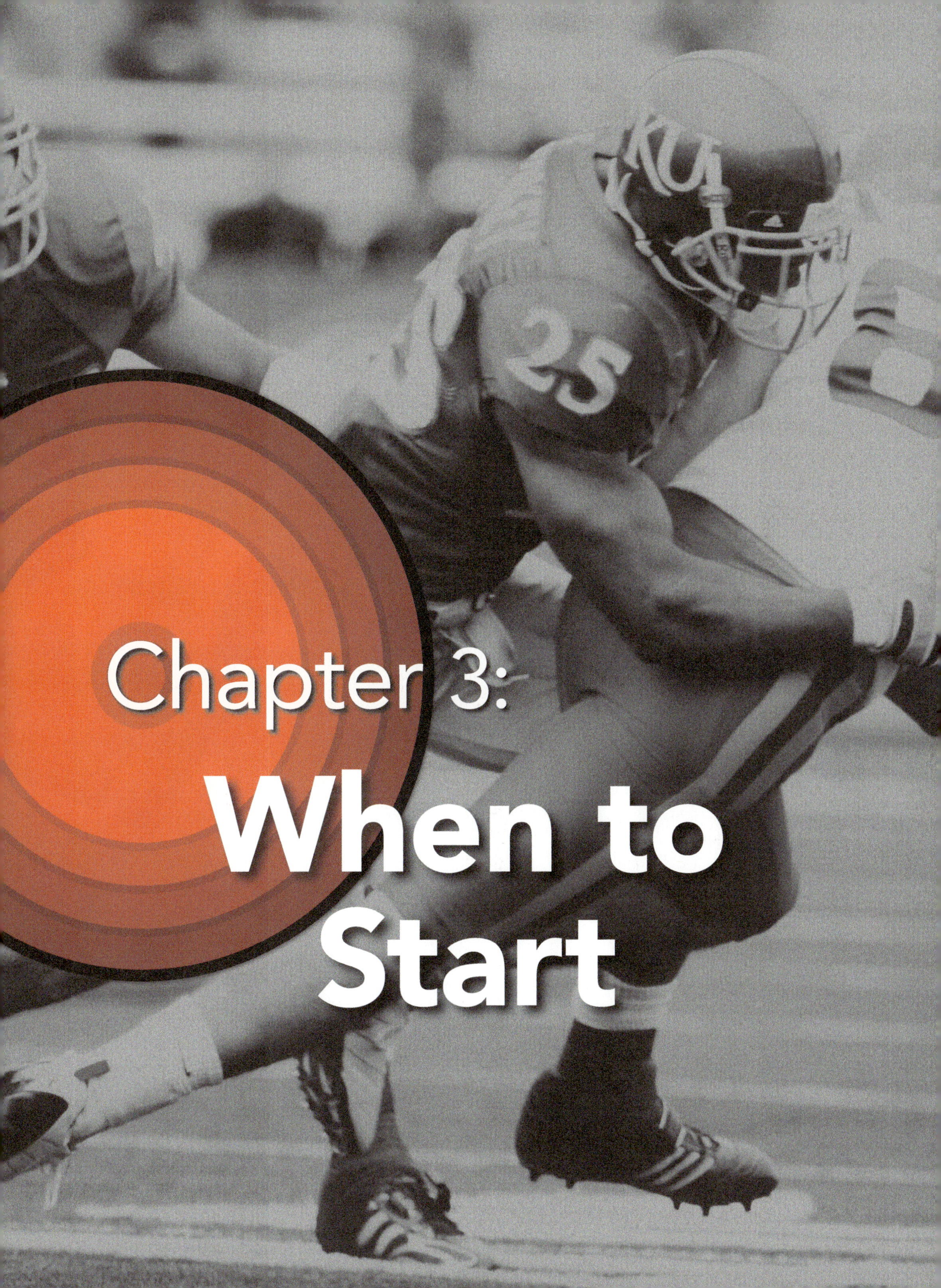

Chapter 3: When to Start

I am often asked by parents and sport coaches to share a year-round performance training program, but it's a hard thing to do. The complicated process of measuring and monitoring athletes and then prescribing workouts to meet their specific goals throughout the year is difficult. It's hard to simply hand someone a workout program without knowing the athlete first. It must be explained that performance is a process, so I immediately direct them to one of the best resources for physical literacy and development, Canadian Sport for Life (www.canadiansportforlife.ca). Canadian Sport for life has a guide for physical development. In this guide, seven different stages for Long-Term Athletic Development (LTAD) are outlined. Each stage is given a name with specific information regarding each developmental stage. The stages range from an active start at birth to active for life after competitive sports.

Sports performance consists of fundamental skills as well as sport specific skills. According to the LTAD guide, fundamental movement skills such as agility, balance, and coordination need to be developed by the age of nine. Kids gallop, skip, run (speed development), and jump (plyometrics) all the time. Formal instruction on these activities should be completed before starting any type of resistance training program. These skills can be refined as a person ages, but a foundation must be developed through physical activity at a young age.

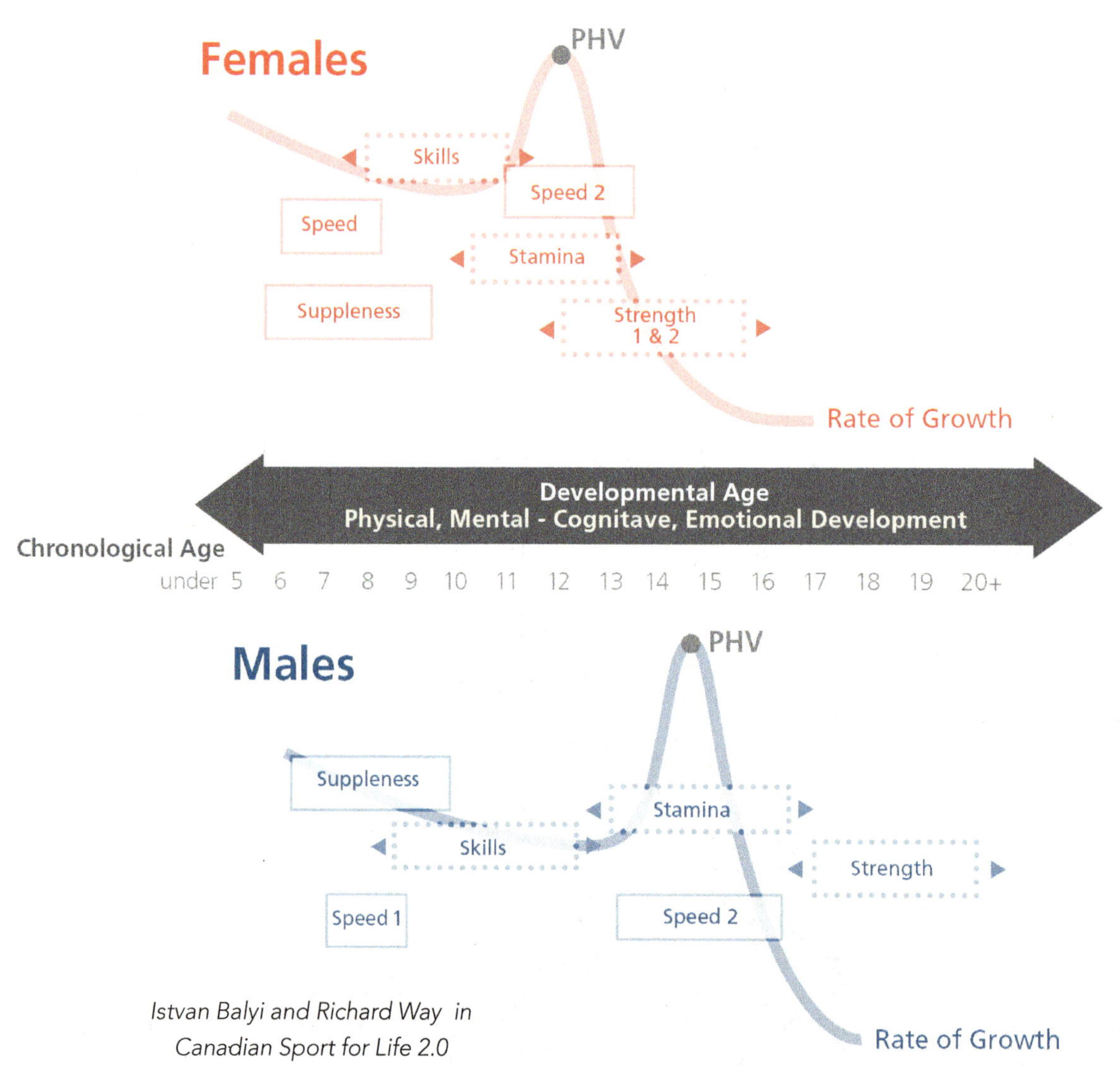

Istvan Balyi and Richard Way in Canadian Sport for Life 2.0

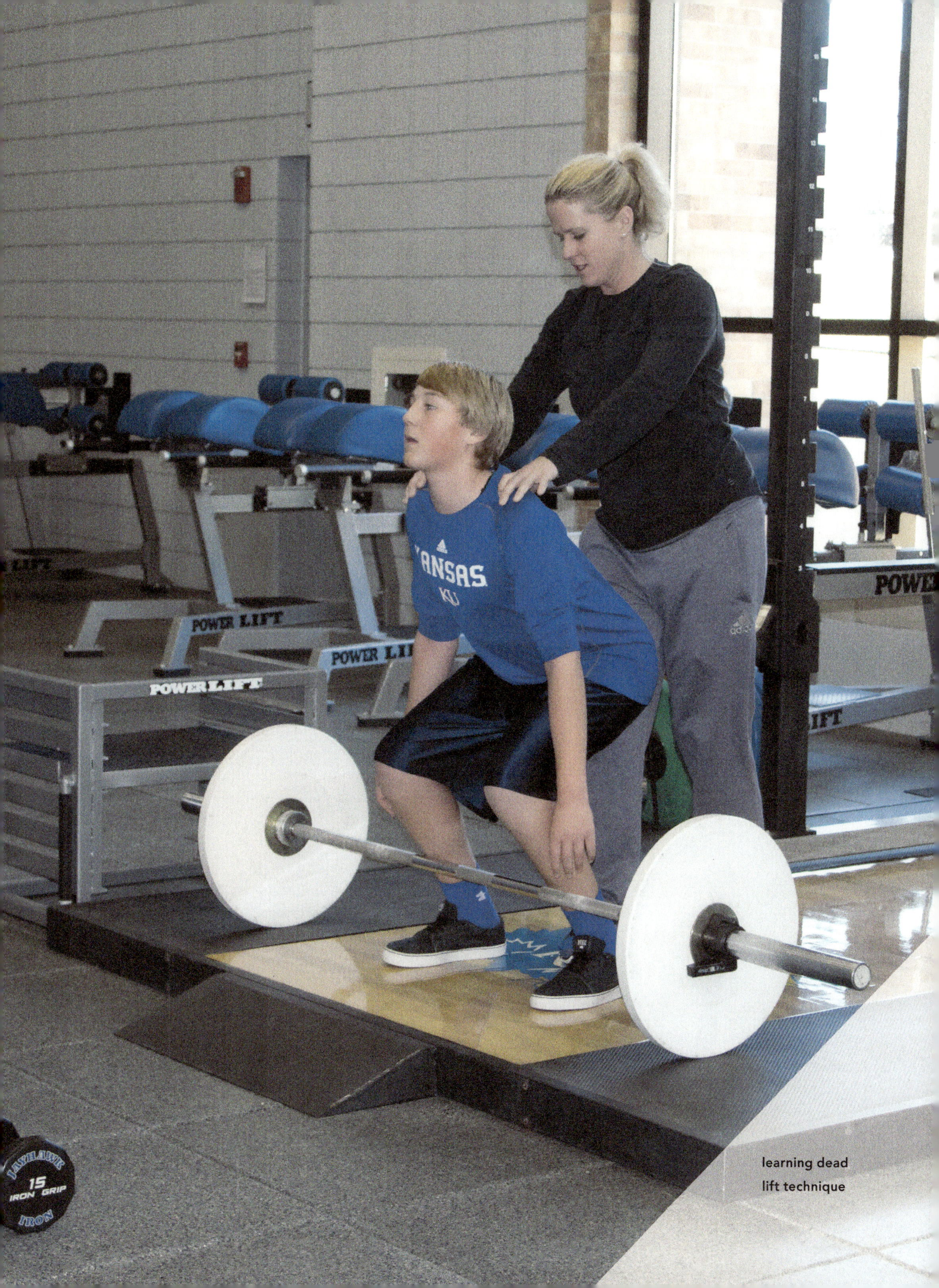

learning dead lift technique

Competition and winning should not be the only focus in youth sports. It should be about progress and development. Specializing in only one or two sports too early may hinder athletic development. The focus should gradually move to specialization and competition as athletes age.

The graph shows a developmental guide for both male and female athletes. The top red graph represents females and the bottom blue graph represents males. Peak Height Velocity (PHV) is defined as the maximum rate of growth during adolescence. This is highlighted because there is a great window for trainability specifically around this time.

There are times when middle school and high school athletes are different in chronological age (age in years), but are the same in developmental age (physical maturity). Coaches need to be aware of the difference between chronological age and developmental age. This is important to note because coaches need to adapt to an athlete's biological age in order to train him/her safely and effectively. It is important for coaches to attend to the specific needs of each individual. If a younger (chronologically) athlete is not as developed as the rest of the team, the coach should adjust that athlete's program to fit his needs. Vice versa, if the athlete is chronologically younger but biologically older, a coach may need to increase the intensity of the workout so the athlete is challenged.

The window of opportunity to optimally strength train females is between twelve to fifteen years and for boys is approximately seventeen. This doesn't mean that one shouldn't strength train before or after this age; it simply shows the optimal time frame to see the greatest benefits. The reason for the difference in age is due to the earlier development in girls as compared to boys.

Understanding where athletes are in their development is extremely important in writing a program. If a program is too advanced, the athlete is at risk for injury. On the contrary, if the program is lacking in volume or intensity, the athlete may not develop properly. By the time an athlete reaches college, the most effective way to gain performance results is through strength training because it is the variable that is closest to PHV.

Listed below are a few questions that need to be taken into consideration before putting an athlete on any type of resistance training program:

1. **What is the developmental age of the athlete?**
2. **What skills does the athlete require?**
3. **Is the athlete healthy?**
4. **Does the athlete want to train?**
5. **What type of program is available?**
6. **What equipment or facilities are available?**
7. **What type of coaching is available?**

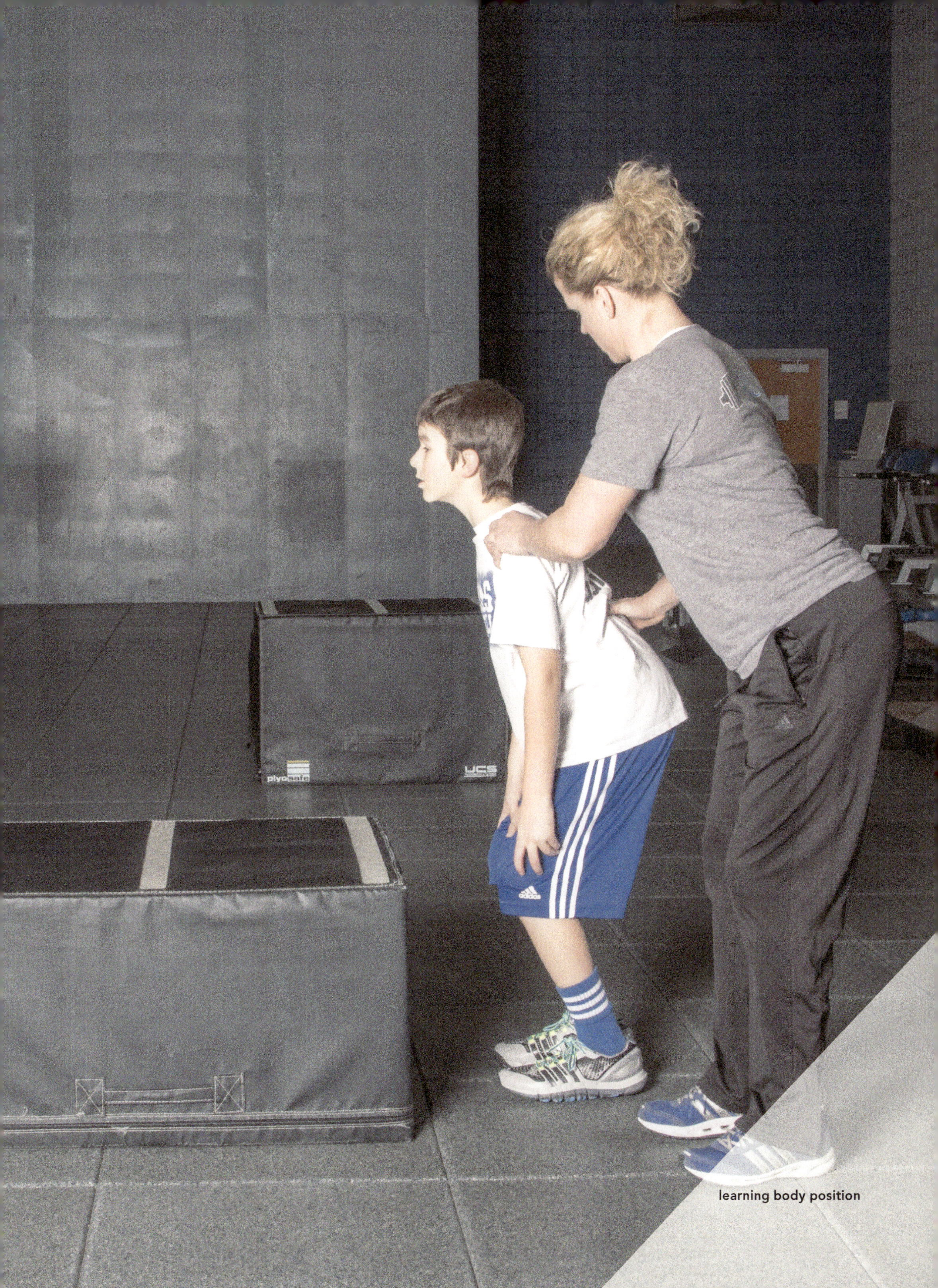

learning body position

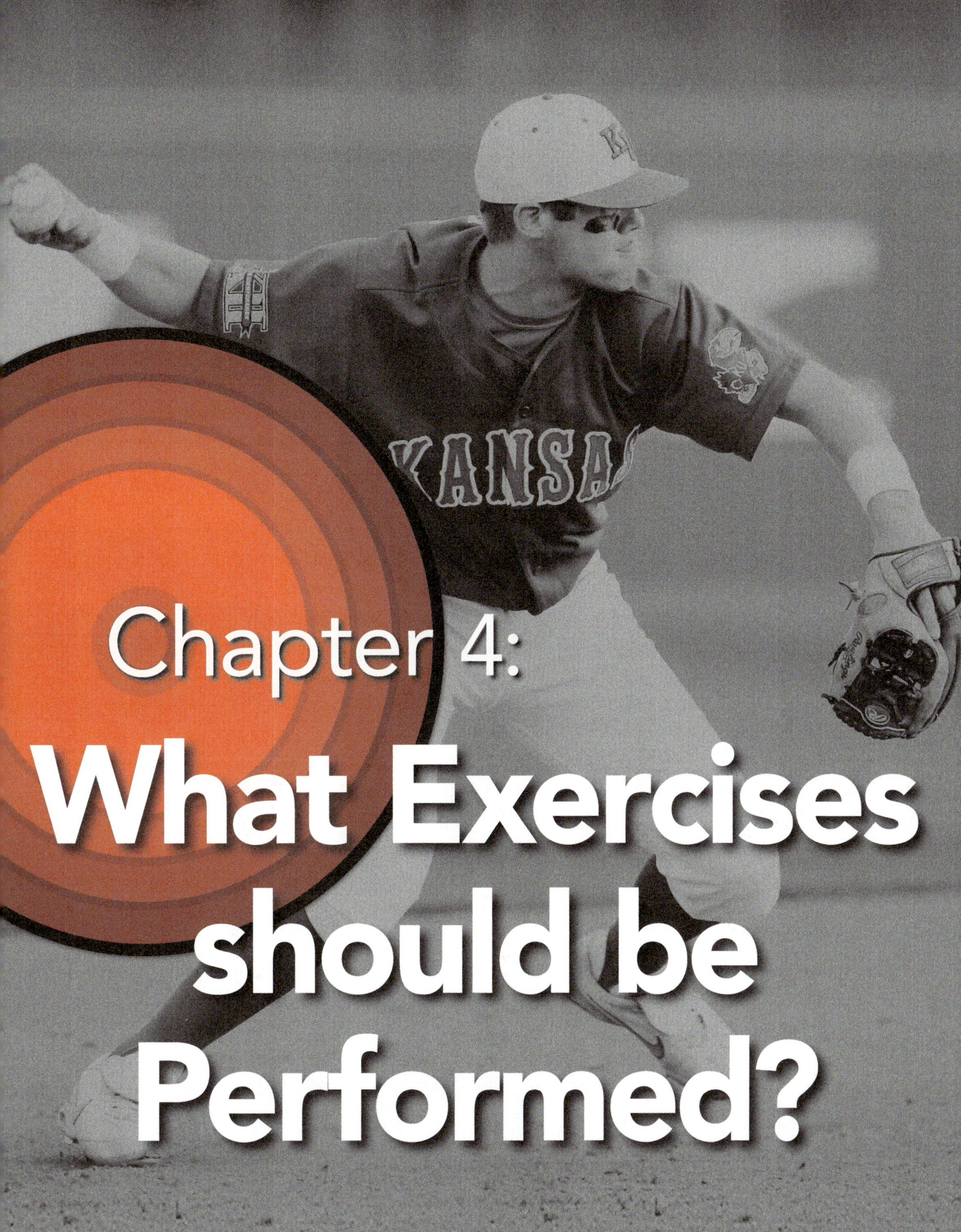

Chapter 4: What Exercises should be Performed?

SECTION 1: Essential Exercises

It is important to establish great movement skills before adding any type of external resistance like free weights. Bodyweight movements and exercises such as walking, running, jumping, squatting, lunging, shuffling, twisting, turning, or any combination thereof should be learned first with skill development and willful intent. Then, if one wants to begin to learn about resistance training with a barbell or dumbbell, use a broomstick or light dumbbells to feel the effects of placement on and around the body. Although these exercises may appear to be easy at first, when done with purpose they can be challenging. Slowly, add external resistance as long as technique is not sacrificed. (Refer to National Strength and Conditioning Association's Strength and Conditioning Journal article on Long-Term Athletic Development and It's Application to Youth Weightlifting by Lloyd, R. S., Oliver, J. L., Meyers, R. W., Moody, J. A. & Stone M. H.)

These are the exercises that one should begin to learn and develop technique:

1. **Explosive exercises that involve speed training, agility training, and plyometrics**
2. **Clean**
3. **Snatch**
4. **Jerk**
5. **Squat**
6. **Dead Lift**
7. **Lunge**
8. **Upper body push**
9. **Upper body pull**

Before anyone prescribes or starts a workout plan, a general understanding of exercise groups and terminology must be reviewed. This is important so everyone is on the same page and you do not waste time defining differences.

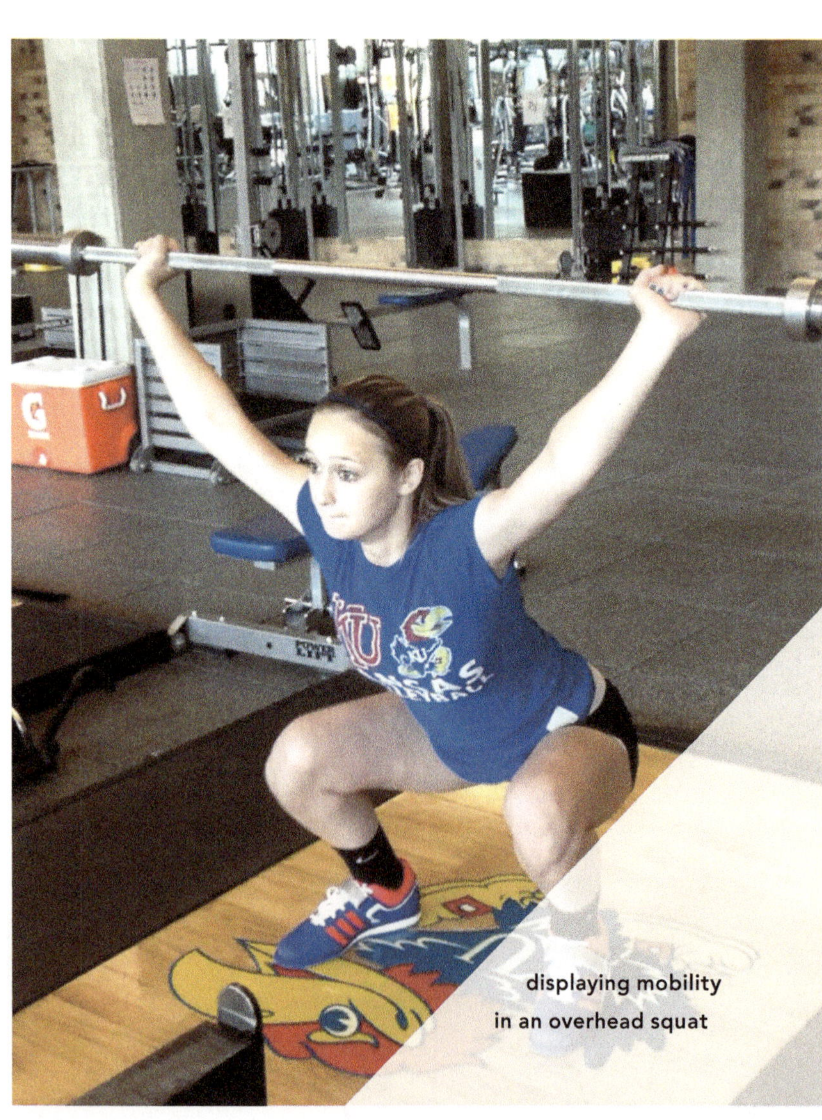

displaying mobility in an overhead squat

WEIGHTIFTING

1. Clean and Jerk
2. Snatch

THE NAME OF THE LIFT DICTATES THE MOVEMENT AND POSITION, THE MOVEMENT AND POSITION DICTATES IT'S PURPOSE

WEIGHTLIFTING VARIATIONS

1. **Hang Clean** – from power position, triple extension, catch with thighs below parallel to the ground
2. **Power Clean** – from floor, triple extension, catch in in a position where the thigh is above parallel to the ground
3. **Hang Power Clean** – from power position, triple extension, catch in a position where the thigh is above parallel to the ground
4. **Split Clean Variations** – catch in split squat position
5. **Hang Snatch** – from power position, triple extension, catch overhead with thighs below parallel to ground
6. **Power Snatch** – from floor, triple extension, catch overhead with thighs above parallel to the ground
7. **Hang Power Snatch** – from power position, triple extension, catch overhead in a position where the thigh is above parallel to the ground
8. **Split Snatch Variations** – catch in a split squat position
9. **Power Jerk** – from a standing position, dip and drive to catch overhead in a position with thighs above parallel to the ground
10. **Split Jerk** – from a standing position, dip and drive to catch overhead in a split squat position
11. **Clean Pull** – from floor, triple extension, arms stay extended
12. **Hi Pull** – from floor, triple extension, then pull the bar to chin with arms bent and elbows above hands

POWERLIFTING

1. Dead Lift
2. Squat
3. Bench

BODY BUILDING

Train for aesthetics or lean mass.
To develop one's musculature.

STRONGMAN COMPETITIONS

Train to display great feats of strength.

RESISTANCE TRAINING

Dumbbells, Kettlebells, Barbells
Water & Manual Resistance
Pneumonic Air Resistance
Medicine Balls
Band Resistance
Selectorized Machines
Plate Loaded Machines
Chains

SECTION 2: Exercise Order

Hopefully, by this point, you can begin to comprehend the complexity and variability of a quality sports performance program. By now you probably understand that a 'one-size fits all program' may not be effective for every athlete on a team. At Kansas University, we can have seventy different workouts with all types of variations for our players throughout the season. If I gave out seventy different workouts to everyone who asked, it could be quite confusing for a coach and the athlete.

The purposes of sports performance training:

1. Increase the rate of force production (speed/reactability)
2. Increase overall quantity of force production-strength (stiffness/compliance)
3. Increase work capacity

Increasing these variables will create a more powerful and efficient athlete. With speed and technique being the primary focus, high-intensity synchronous movements should always precede the lower intensity asynchronous movements.

Types of Exercises:

SYNCHRONOUS - Muscle recruitment at the same time for power. In sync.

ASYNCHRONOUS – Muscle recruitment at different times for endurance. Not in sync.

Synchronous	Asynchronous
High intensity	Low intensity
High Power	High Endurance
Clean	Circuit Training
Max Vertical Jump	Jump rope
Acceleration	Marathon
Agility	Jogging

The reason synchronous exercises should be completed first is because you never want to train speed, acceleration, agility, or power when the central nervous system (CNS) is in a fatigued state. If you are training to become more explosive and/or quicker, this is extremely important.

Understand that there is a difference between CNS fatigue and muscle fatigue. An example of muscular fatigue is performing a lift until you can no longer complete another repetition. This is called momentary muscular fatigue. When your CNS is fatigued, you can still physically complete the lift, however, movement velocity is compromised. When it comes to the human body we have to remember that the body adapts to the stress that is put on it. If you train slowly, the body will adapt by becoming slower. This is the main reason we do not do sets of 20 repetitions of power or weightlifting movements. Arguably, beyond five repetitions, barbell velocity begins to significantly slow down.

One of the purposes of weightlifting is to increase the rate of force development (improve the rate at which the muscles are able to develop high levels of force). Physically this can be done, but to perform a high amount of repetitions of these exercises in a row will simply not train speed. Speed of movement diminishes as the repetitions get higher. This is the main drawback to many popular training programs such as Insanity, Crossfit, P90X, etc. Those workouts are tough, make you sweat, and force you to work hard; however, if you are truly training to improve speed and quickness, completing high volume sets of CNS fatiguing activities is actually going to do the opposite for you.

Asynchronous activities are movements that do not stress the CNS as much and therefore, as a general rule, should be completed after all synchronous activities. The purpose of these movements or lifts is not necessarily to increase the rate of force development which is why they can be done while in a CNS fatigued state.

The intensity of the exercise can be dictated by either the load (how much weight is lifted) or the speed of movement (how fast you lift it). Remember to focus on technique and always progress gradually.

Below is a percentage chart that we have adopted to fit our scenario at Kansas University. As athletes begin to progress with external resistance, we use these basic guidelines for loading, reps, and goals. All exercises are different and loading schemes can vary from exercise to exercise and athlete to athlete.

Hypertrophy	Strength-Speed	Strength	Speed-Strength
Moderate Velocity (long healthy compliant contractions)	**High Velocity** (maximum intent, ballistic contractions)	**Moderate Velocity** (maximum intent, compliant contraction)	**High Velocity** (maximum intent, ballistic contractions)
8-10-12 reps	**1-5 reps**	**6-8 reps**	**3-6 reps**
60-76% of max	85-91% of max	76-85% of max	60-90% of max

Fleck, S.J., and W.J. Kraemer. *Designing Resistance Training Programs.* Champaign, IL: Human Kinetics. 1987. Print Siff, Mel. *Supertraining.* Denver, CO: Supertraining Institute. 2004. Print

Chapter 5:

How to Program

SECTION 1: Periodization

When I first started working with Olympic sport coaches and athletes at the University of Connecticut, planning and scheduling weight room time was not a priority; logically, the on-court/field practice was the priority. Anytime I was given access to the athletes, I jumped at the opportunity. I would gather them into the weight room to get them to perform any type of training they were motivated to do. Sometimes they were fatigued after practice and sometimes they were fresh before practice. In such cases, the coach allowed them to lift before practice or a simple 'walk-thru' practice was only performed prior. There was no consistency to the training schedule. The athlete's ability to produce power on a day-to-day basis was not consistent because of the rigorous practice and game schedules. The only thing that was consistent was the inconsistency.

I would often consult with my colleagues about my frustrations of not having enough time to properly train the athletes. The coaches had trouble seeing and making the skill sets of performance training a priority. I was fortunate enough to have my office close to a world-renowned research scientist in resistance training and exercise, Dr. William Kraemer. I consulted with him daily. We often talked about the battle to develop a consistent training program for coaches and athletes who did not want to make sports performance training a priority. Dr. Kraemer looked at it differently. With his vast experiences of being an athlete, coach, and research scientist, he suggested that I adapt to them. I was confused at first. Adapt to them? I was hesitant because I was taught that in order to have a training effect, we had to either have a separate weight training session earlier in the day or at the start of practice (and there were very few coaches at the time who would even let me present that as an option). Dr. Kraemer convinced me that with a variable and adaptable training program we may be able to develop a results-based program with minimal time commitment and planning.

So that is what I did. I was able to create a program that adapted to everyone else's schedule. I was constantly communicating with the coaches and athletes about goals, overall state of athletic readiness, and fatigue levels. Every day was different. If the games or practices were good, everyone had a great attitude and was willing to do what I asked of them in the weight room. If the games and practices were bad, it was a lot harder to get the training affect that was needed, but we still completed workouts and gained results. This is why we use flexible and non-flexible non-linear periodization (NLP) throughout the year.

The loading scheme (how much weight is used during an exercise or training session) can change on a day-to-day, week-to-week, month-to-month basis.

Non-linear periodization (NLP) is planning and adjusting the following:

1. **Load** - how much weight you lift
2. **Volume** - how many reps, sets, pounds, etc. you completed
3. **Intensity** - your effort in simple terms of high, medium, and low/throughout your program

I use NLP because of its variability. The workout is based on how an individual feels and performs on a certain day. Basically during the week, one can train the neuromuscular (nervous and muscle) system to increase muscular power (1 - 6 reps). Power can be trained two different ways: One day you can focus on heavier weight (strength/speed) and the other day you can focus on lighter weight at a faster speed (speed/strength). Another day can simply be a strength (reps 1-8) day. The fourth day one can train the body's biochemical (cardiovascular and chemical) system to increase muscular endurance (high reps 10-12).

This is completely different from linear periodization programs where one begins with higher volume and lower load programs and ends with lower volume and heavier load programs after months of training. Linear periodization programs are great for people who have a set schedule and routine in their life. There is less variability in terms of volume and load throughout the week and month. This type of programming does not change on a daily basis.

There are two types of non-linear periodization:

1. Planned Non-linear Periodization- when the days can be planned ahead of time and the competition and sport practice schedule is secondary to training. This is done outside of competitive season.
2. Flexible Non-linear Periodization - When the workouts are not planned and are based on the athlete's physical and mental state. This is done in the competitive season.

PLANNED NON-LINEAR PERIODIZATION

The following is a simple way to look at a general repetition plan for four days/week for three months.

MONTH 1

	Workout #1	Workout #2	Workout #3	Workout #4
REPS	**8-10-12**	**1-5**	**6-8**	**3-6**
GOAL	Muscle Hypertrophy	Muscle Power (strength/speed)	Muscle Strength	Muscle Power (speed/strength)

MONTH 2

In the second month the repetitions can change with a linear periodization trend by slightly decreasing volume and increasing loads each training day.

	Workout #1	Workout #2	Workout #3	Workout #4
REPS	**10**	**1-4**	**7**	**3-6**
GOAL	Muscle Hypertrophy	Muscle Power (strength/speed)	Muscle Strength	Muscle Power (speed/strength)

MONTH 3

After the second month, the training 'plan' can be re-evaluated. If the coach feels that it is appropriate, the athlete should be able continue to increase loads in month three.

	Workout #1	Workout #2	Workout #3	Workout #4
REPS	**10-12**	**1-3**	**6**	**3-5**
GOAL	Muscle Hypertrophy	Muscle Power (strength/speed)	Muscle Strength	Muscle Power (speed/strength)

After three months of training, one's competitive season may be starting. The training needs to adapt to the skill development and conditioning that occur primarily for what you are training for. So, the training program then switches to flexible non-linear periodization.

FLEXIBLE NON-LINEAR PERIODIZATION

MONTH 4

As your training progresses, the muscle endurance/work capacity/conditioning that was occurring in the weight room is replaced by the conditioning that is occurring on the court/field/track during practice. The focus in the weight room then becomes maintaining strength and increasing power and speed.

	Workout #1	Workout #2	Workout #3
REPS	**1-2**	**6-8**	**3-4**
GOAL	Muscle Power (strength/speed)	Muscle Strength	Muscle Power (speed/strength)

The beauty of this plan is that the days are in no particular order. The schedule is adaptable. If an individual is feeling great, focused, and full of energy about 3 hours after he wakes up or at lunchtime, he can perform a workout requiring technique that can increase power, strength, and speed on any day of the week. This workout would involve high load and low reps. If he trains after work and he is feeling tired and unfocused, he can perform a workout that can still have an effect. A high volume circuit in machines or free weights is an example of training the biochemical system to increase muscular endurance. This will help you increase your metabolism and burn fat. Although, if he/she feels good after practice or work, by all means lift heavy.

So, you could have a weekly schedule that looks like this:

	Workout #1	Workout #2	Workout #3	Workout #4
REPS	3-5	6	1-3	10-12
GOAL	Muscle Power (speed/strength)	Muscle Strength	Muscle Power (strength/speed)	Muscle Hypertrophy

Basically, on days the individual feels good, use more weight to elicit a strength response or move faster to receive a power response. On days the individual doesn't feel as good, do something, like a simple circuit (lower loads, more reps). But make sure that on any training day that the individual completes some type of workout.

Non-linear programs are great for athletes because practice may get in the way of the training schedule. Also, non-linear programs are great for anyone who wants to train because life just gets in the way!

Each workout session should start with some type of warm up. The specific exercises that you do in your warm up depend upon the workout for that day. For example, if you are going to bench press, you may want to include push ups and/or some shoulder stabilization exercises before you load up the bar and begin pressing it. If you are going to squat, then performing some bodyweight squats would be a good idea to do beforehand. If the session is a speed/strength day and has a lot of plyometrics, then warm up with some low level plyometrics such as an agility ladder or a jump rope.

While your options for warming up vary greatly, there are a few principles to keep in mind. First, the warm up should be designed to increase your heart rate as well as to begin delivering oxygenated blood to the muscles that are going to be trained during the workout. Your warm up is also a great place to work on flexibility, mobility and individual areas in need of improvement. Generally speaking, ten to fifteen minutes should be enough time to properly warm up the body.

After you warm up, the next part of the workout should involve the activities that stress your central nervous system (CNS) the most. This would include plyometrics, movement mechanics or agility work, any weightlifting movements, or explosive lifts that are designed to improve power output.

Evaluation of yourself and your training regimen is extremely important – are you seeing results? Do you need to change something? Are you successful? Why or why not? As stated previously, there is nothing wrong with failing, as long as you understand why and then work to improve it.

Workouts should be consistently completed every week. Our success at Kansas is based on our commitment to a 46-48 week per year program. Those days/weeks/months add up to a lot of reps. Our lives are about quality reps.

SECTION 2: Before You Start

As athletes, coaches, and parents, you are all too familiar with the annual "physical" that must be completed before athletes are allowed to participate. Although sometimes this seems like just another task to take off of the "to do" list, it is actually one of the most important steps that needs to be taken before any training program begins.

The information gained from general pre-participation physicals, including personal and family medical history, is invaluable and necessary for maintaining good health and preventing further illness and injury.

Discussion points with the physician, parent, athlete, and coach are not limited to, but should include:

- Previous injuries, illness, existing medical concerns
- Current medications and potential side-effects of that medication while under intense physical exertion
- Family history of cardiovascular disease and potential risk with genetic predisposition
- Exercise induced respiratory difficulties or distress

Additional screenings that are recommended and should be considered before vigorous exercise are: Pre-season baseline concussion testing, EKG/cardiovascular exams, and screenings for blood disorders such as sickle cell, etc.

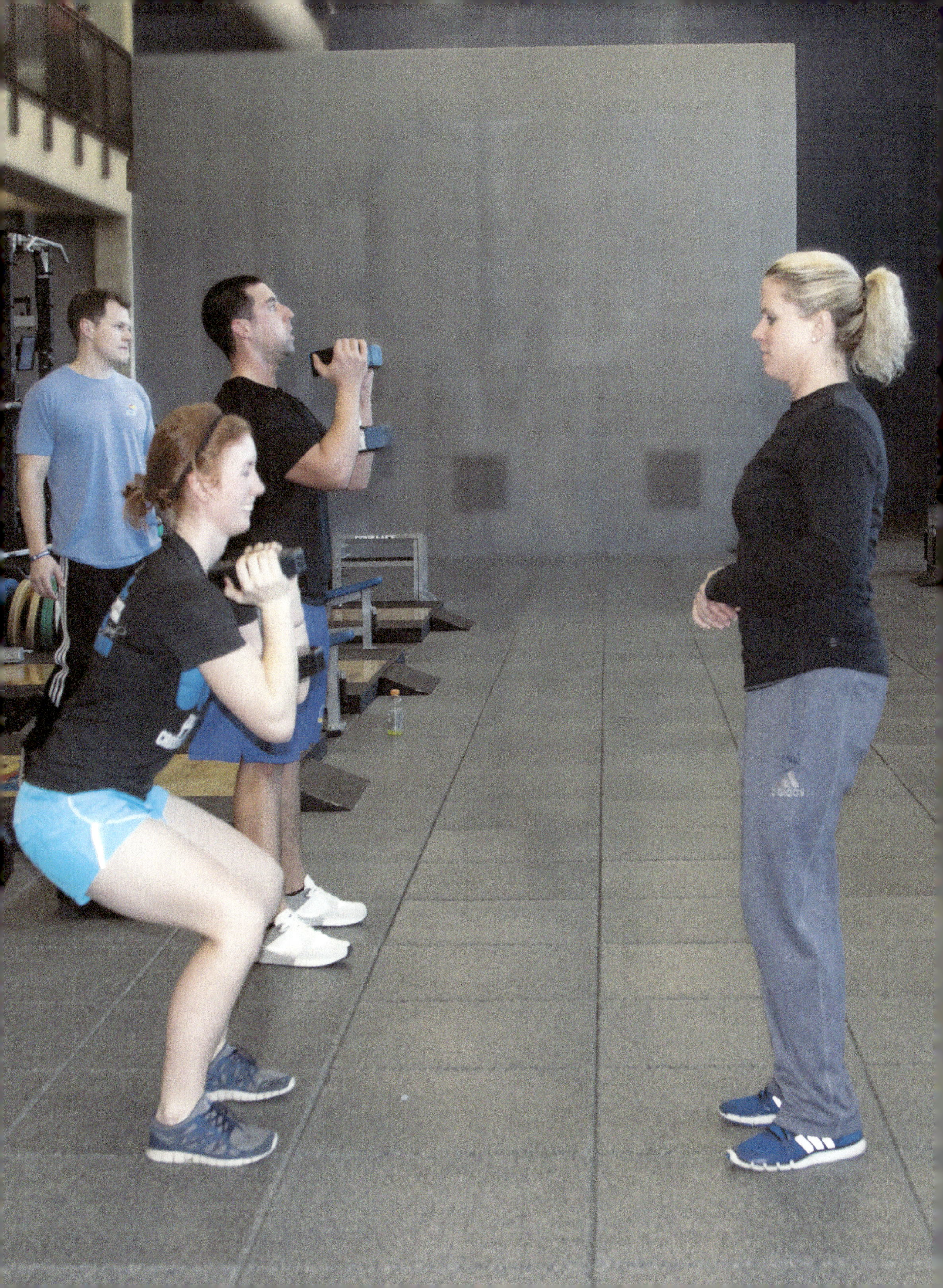

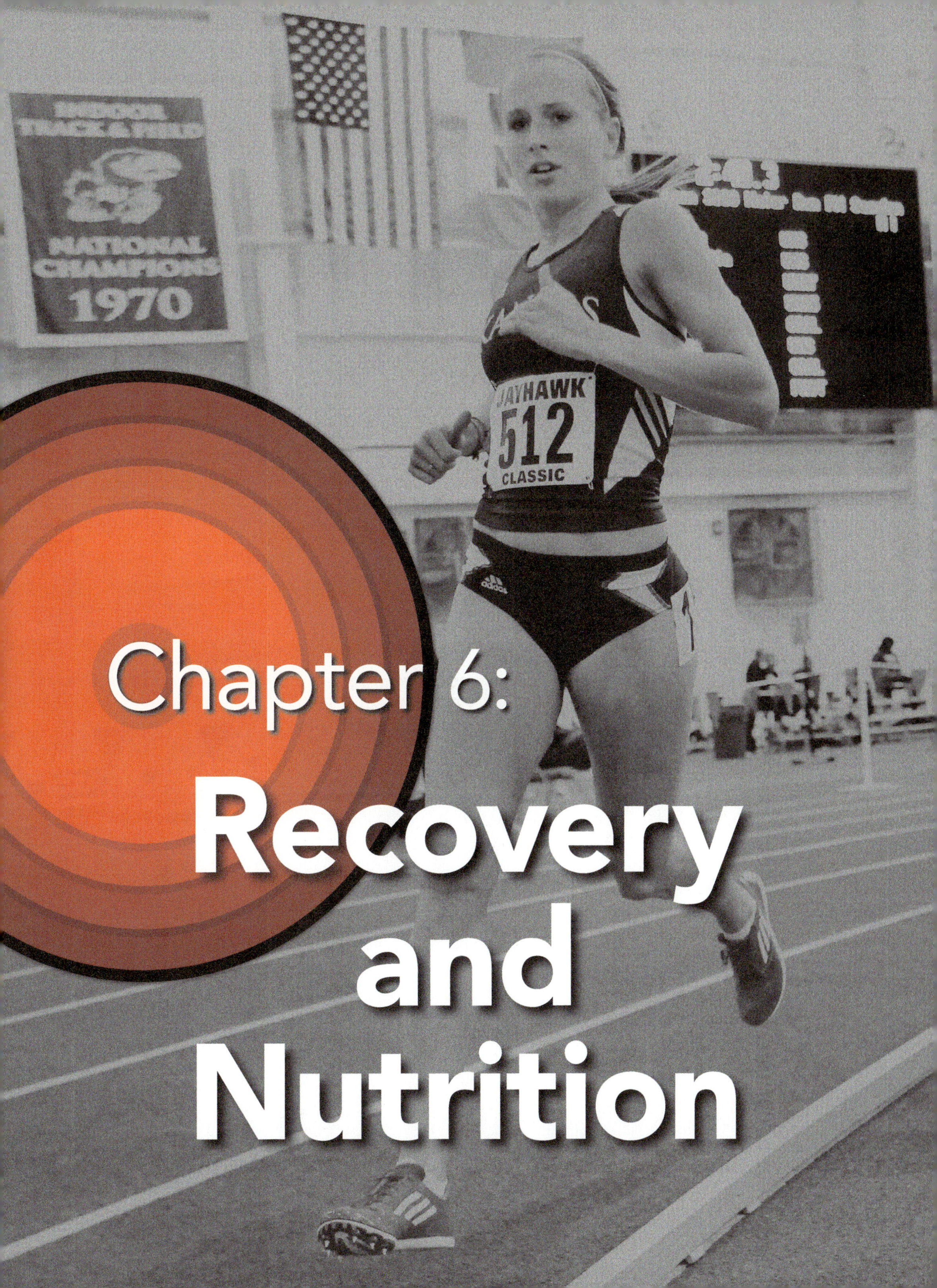

Chapter 6: Recovery and Nutrition

SECTION 1: Recovery

Recovery skills are important and should be utilized year-around. They become exceptionally important when an athlete is in-season because of the increased time and work committed to preparing for competition. Recovery skills significantly decrease the chances of injury and increase performance.

Our recovery program addresses the following:

- Soft tissue manipulation
- Compression
- Sleep health
- Nutrition education

Dr. Phil Wagner of Sparta Sports Science gave us the idea to provide assembled bags and resources that are readily available to each athlete. Many of the items in the bag are reused sports balls or cheaper items that we can get at a home store. The bag has the athlete's number on the front and is designed to be carried while traveling. Each recovery bag contains one of the following that addresses different aspects of recovery:

- PVC pipe
- Tennis, golf, and lacrosse balls
- Nutrition tips
- Compression sleeves
- Rope
- Neck pillows
- Earplugs
- Eye masks
- Sleep monitors

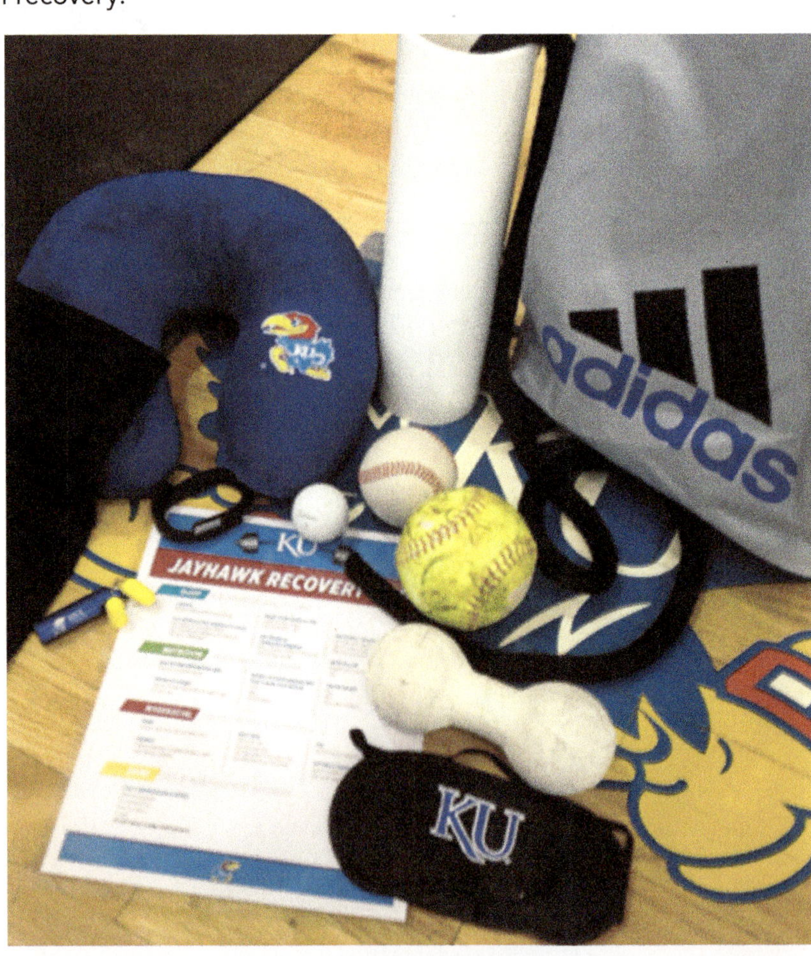

SOFT TISSUE MANIPULATION

We begin teaching soft tissue manipulation techniques as soon as the athlete starts to train. Using the PVC pipe, foam roller or various sized balls, we perform soft tissue manipulations to break up adhesions and increase blood flow to an area. This should make a muscle more compliant so it glides easier to make movement more efficient. Soft tissue manipulation techniques are part of our general warm-up and/or to release specific areas based on an athlete's Sparta scan. For example, with our highly stiff and reactive athletes, we target the calves, hip flexors, IT bands, adductors, and parts of the trunk in order to release stiffness that may be detrimental to the athlete's health.

The travel schedule is often times rigorous and can affect the body. The cramped space of the buses and airplanes, packing, unpacking, interrupted sleep patterns, and various hotel nuances all take their toll. Travel can increase an athlete's stiffness and make them uncomfortable. Being seated in a flexed position for hours at a time can affect muscle length and compliance. Soft tissue manipulation techniques can assist in increasing muscle compliance and movement to help the athlete feel and move better.

COMPRESSION

Research completed by Dr. William Kraemer shows that athletes who wear compression sleeves improve recovery even while at rest. Compression sleeves that contain 24-28% Lycra increase venous and lymphatic return. Increased flow can facilitate soft tissue repair by immobilizing muscle fibers to decrease swelling and regulate fluid buildup inside the body. Dr. Kraemer's research found that the sleeve helps during movement by improving stability and reducing the oscillatory movement of muscle when impacting the ground during running and jumping.

As a result, we provide compression sleeves as a part of our recovery system. Athletes are encouraged to take advantage of these during performance activities and after workouts or games. We emphasize use of the compression sleeves especially during those non-active states such as travel, while sleeping, and during classes.

SLEEP HEALTH

While visiting Sparta Science in Menlo Park, CA, I had to the opportunity to meet Dr. Cheri Mah, a sleep researcher at the University of Stanford Sleep Laboratory. She shared some great research and insights regarding sleep, recovery, and performance.

Healthy sleep helps the following:

1. **Physical recovery**
2. **Increases energy and focus**
3. **Helps motor function**
4. **Decreases injury risk**
5. **Helps metabolism**
6. **Increases reaction time**

We made it a priority to monitor sleep and teach our athletes about the benefits of the quantity and quality of sleep. Dr. Cheri Mah recommended the following:

1. **Payback sleep debt**
2. **Get eight to ten hours**
3. **Take a nap between 1-4pm for no longer than 20-30 min.**
4. **Develop a sleep routine**
5. **Avoid spicy, fried, and tomato based foods before bed**
6. **Create a sleep environment**
    - **No noise**
    - **No sunlight**
    - **65 degrees**

SECTION 2: Nutrition Education

Aaron Carbuhn MS/MS, RD, CSSD, SCCC

The University of Kansas Sports Nutritionist, Aaron Carbuhn, provides the following framework and guidelines that we use to educate our athletes. The field of performance nutrition can sometimes be difficult to comprehend and interpret into real world applications. Even though the schedule is non-traditional and rigorous, building a championship diet and good habits can be easier than you might believe. Just like with any sport there are fundamentals that you must master in order to be successful. This is no different with nutrition. Simply master the following performance nutrition fundamentals DAILY and take your game to the next level!

Eat a Balanced Breakfast

As shown, a balanced breakfast should include protein, fruit, and fats. Additional food sources such as grains/starches and vegetables are encouraged when weight gain is desired or training intensity/volume is high in efforts to better support recovery, energy levels, and boost immune function. See the breakfast food examples above and build a balanced performance breakfast today.

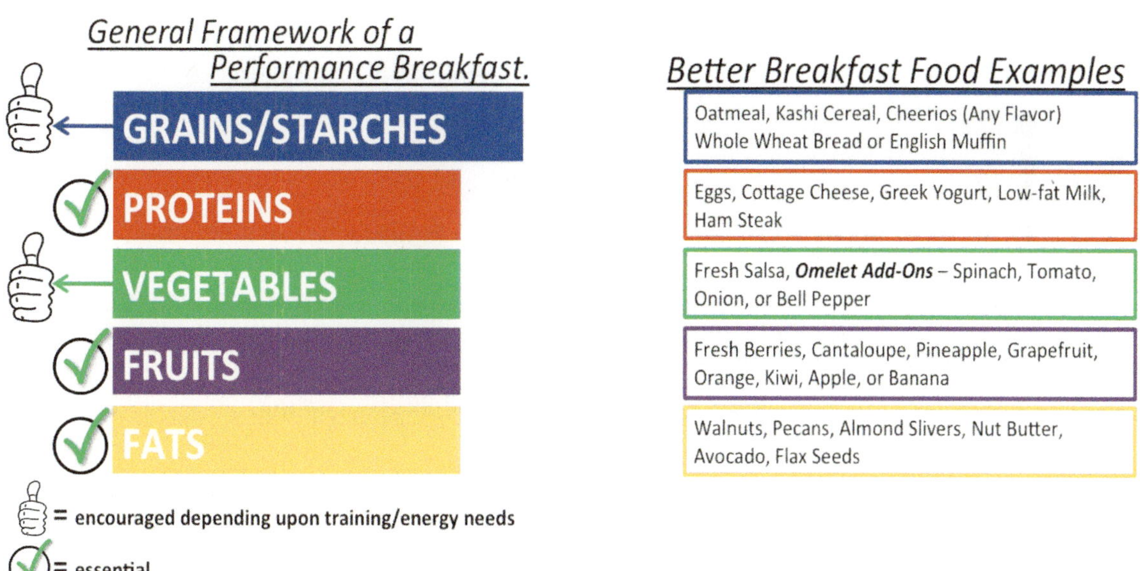

Refrain From Back-loading Your Calories

Back-loading calories refers to consuming the bulk of your calories at the end of the day. Too often athletes get too caught up in their busy schedule and forget to adequately fuel their body during the day for practice/training. This approach will likely result in choosing poorer food choices at dinner which if practiced consistently can decrease performance. Aim for eating approximately half of your daily energy needs by lunch or mid-afternoon. This will not only help fuel training, but also prevent overconsumption at the end of the day.

Hydrate Early and Often

Too often inadequate hydration throughout the day and around training is a primary reason for performance decrements.

Minimum Daily Hydration Prescription
1/2 of body weight (lbs) in fluid oz.

Performance Hydration Framework:

Urine can be a great indicator of hydration status. The urine chart above will help provide you insight on if your current hydration routine is sufficient to support high level training. An easy remedy to improving/meeting your daily hydration prescription is having a water bottle handy at all times. Build a routine of sipping predominately water throughout the day. Do not necessarily rely just on your thirst sensation. More often when you become thirsty you are already dehydrated. Not a good thing when trying to boost training intensity and overall athletic performance.

Hydration Time Frame:	Fluid Ounces of Water:
2 hr - 3hr Before	16 - 24 fl oz
30 Minutes Before	5 - 10 fl oz
Every 15-20 Minutes During Practice or Training Session	5 - 10 fl oz
Immediately After Practice/Training Session	17-20 fl oz per pound lost

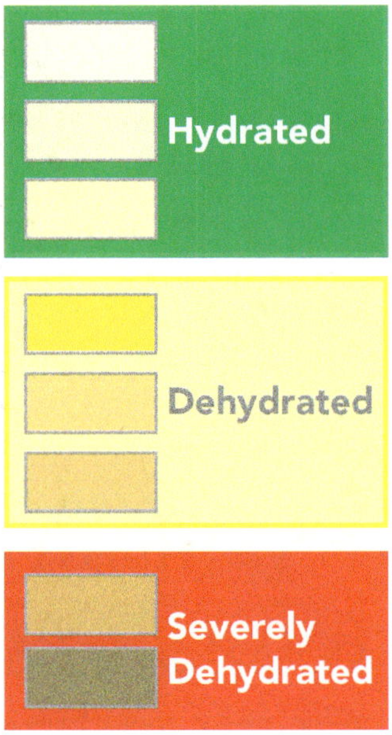

Hydrated

Dehydrated

Severely Dehydrated

Don't Drink Your Calories.... That Includes Alcohol

Too often without realizing many athletes consume a good portion of their daily caloric intake from what they drink. For example, juice, sports drink outside of training, soda, sweet tea, and alcohol. All of these fluids consumed in excess will disrupt energy levels, cause sleep disturbances, and over time can cause a gain of unwanted body fat which could decrease athletic performance. Stick to calorie free fluids. Consume your calories from food and keep these fluid calories to a minimum, especially alcohol!

Snack Smart – Bedtime Included

Be smart with your snack options. Keep your snack foods as nutrient dense as possible and refrain from choosing typical snack options with empty calories. Snacks should be balanced with your choice of either a protein or fat coupled with a fruit or vegetable. This will provide the energy any athlete needs to power through the day.

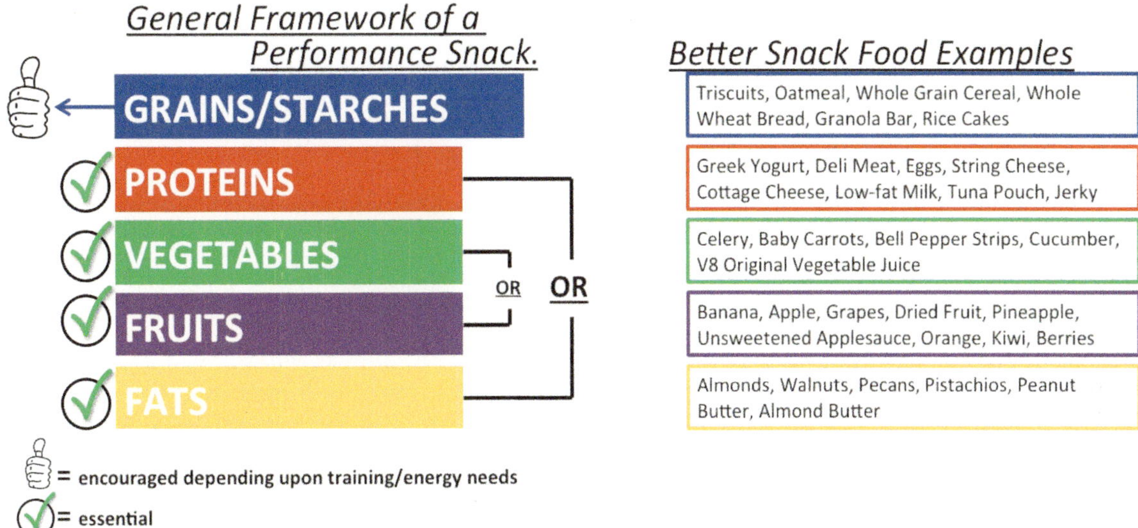

Don't Skip Recovery Nutrition

Proper nutrition within 30-60 minutes after training is crucial in the recovery process. Recovery nutrition will help repair and build muscle as well as replace depleted energy levels. This will allow your body to attack tomorrow's workout with the same high intensity. Therefore, view recovery nutrition as building for tomorrow. After hard training sessions look to consume between 10-30g of protein and at least 50g of carbohydrates. For example, low-fat chocolate and a piece of fresh fruit would easily meet the protein and carbohydrate requirements. For additional ideas please see the general framework below. If looking to add more weight or in need of additional carbohydrates due to high training volume/frequency look to add additional grain options to your plan.

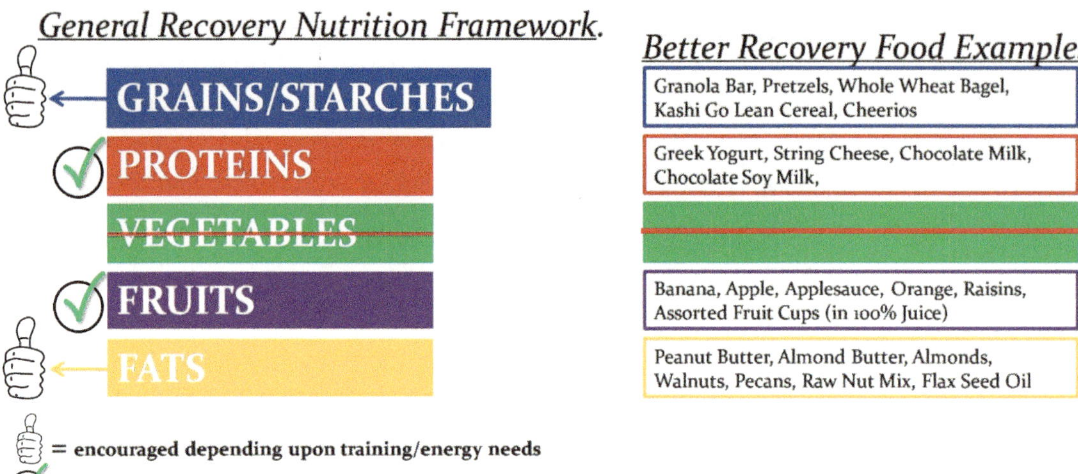

Know Your Dinner Performance Plates

Many athletes find themselves fueling their body the same at dinner regardless of how they trained that day. The performance plates below will help guide you on how to build your plate according to your training day. Nutrition should be adjusted when training is altered. Simply follow the plate outline with the appropriate hand specific serving sizes. Your body and training will thank you.

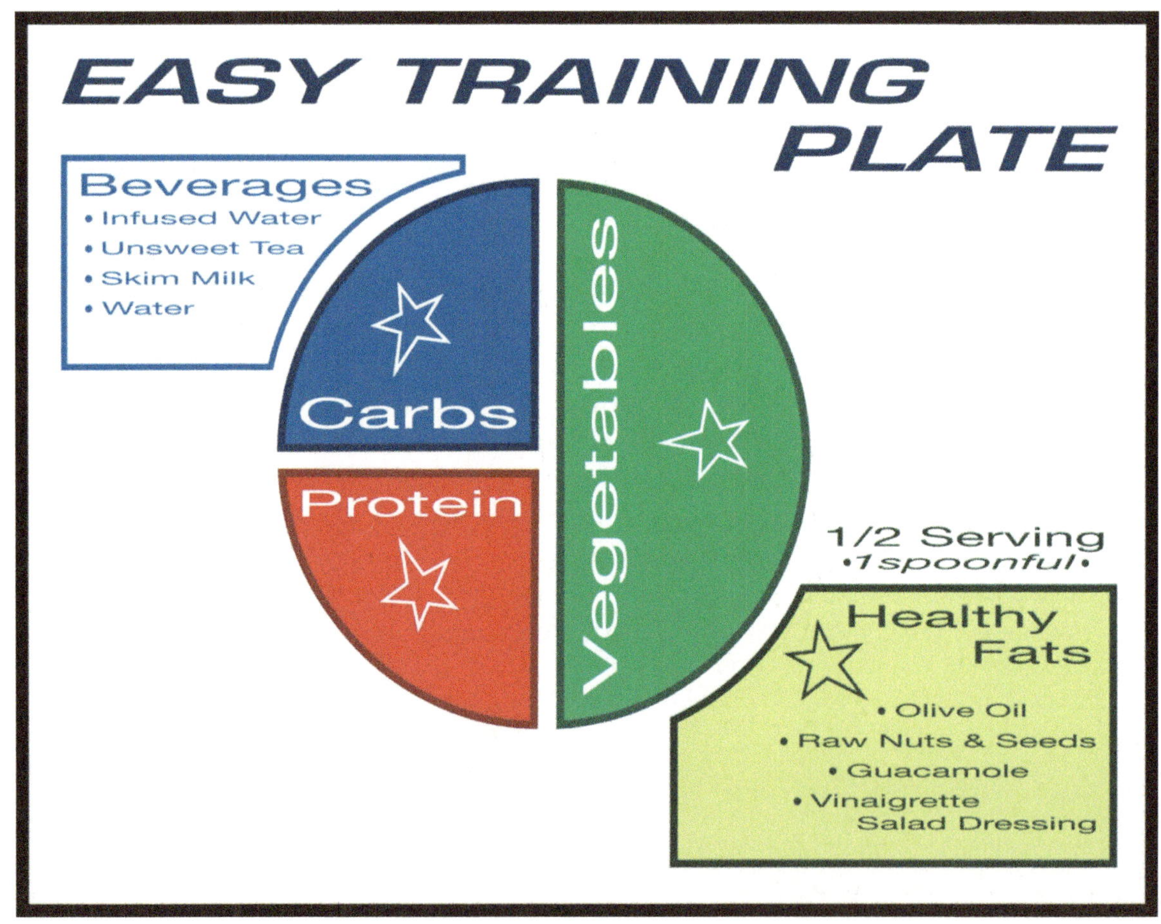

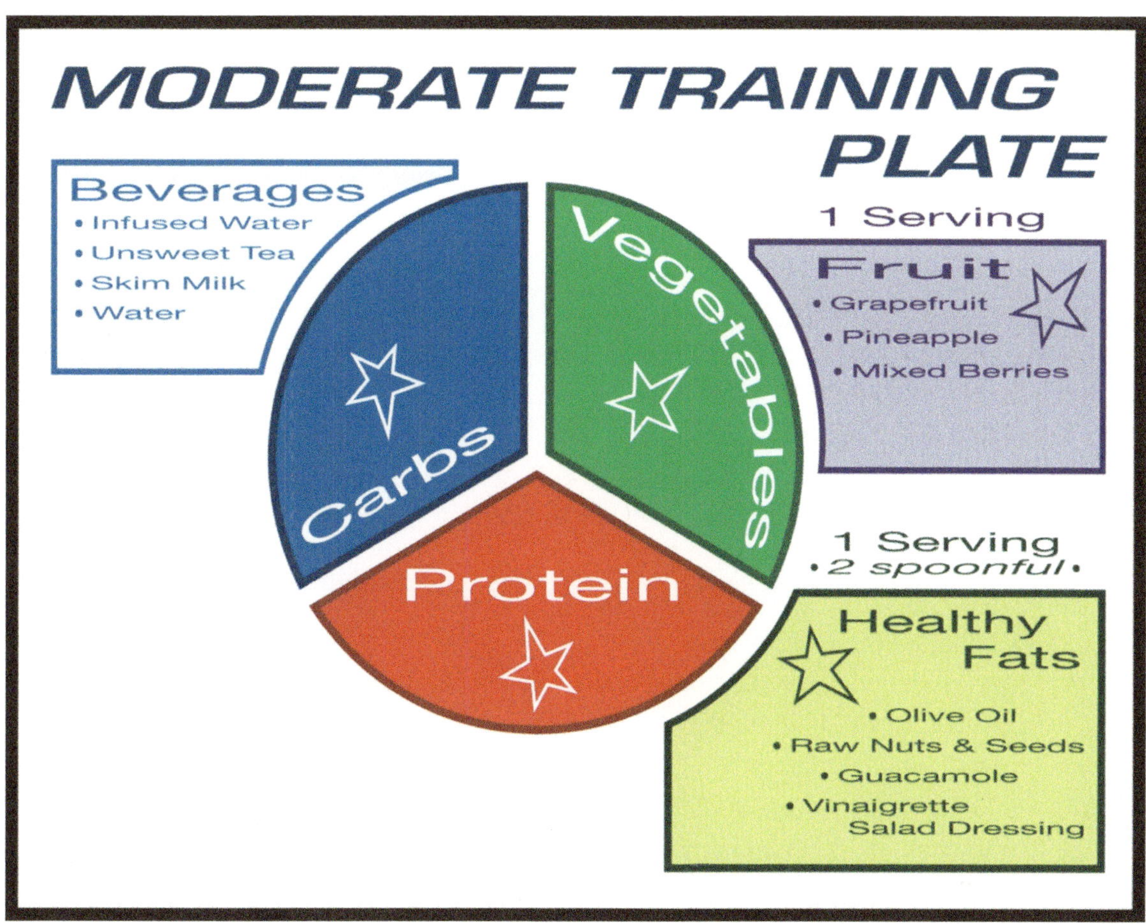
MODERATE TRAINING PLATE
Beverages
• Infused Water
• Unsweet Tea
• Skim Milk
• Water
Carbs
Vegetables
Protein
1 Serving
Fruit
• Grapefruit
• Pineapple
• Mixed Berries
1 Serving
•2 spoonful•
Healthy Fats
• Olive Oil
• Raw Nuts & Seeds
• Guacamole
• Vinaigrette Salad Dressing

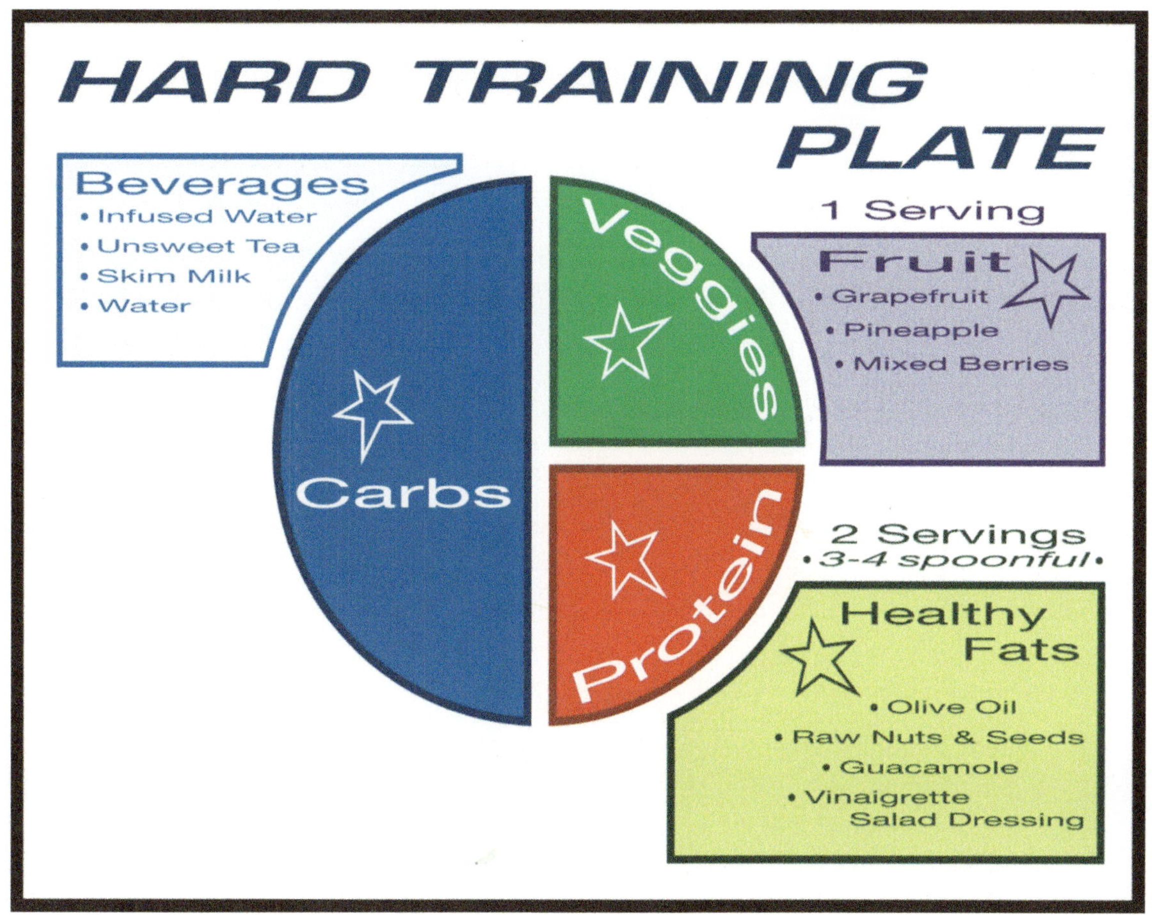
HARD TRAINING PLATE
Beverages
• Infused Water
• Unsweet Tea
• Skim Milk
• Water
Carbs
Veggies
Protein
1 Serving
Fruit
• Grapefruit
• Pineapple
• Mixed Berries
2 Servings
•3-4 spoonful•
Healthy Fats
• Olive Oil
• Raw Nuts & Seeds
• Guacamole
• Vinaigrette Salad Dressing